FROM

HOT

Mess

to

Happiness

FROM HOT MESS TO HAPPINESS

2023 YGTMedia Co. Press Trade Paperback Edition.

Copyright @ 2023 Heather Lind

Published in Canada, for Global Distribution by YGTMedia Co.

www.ygtmedia.co

For more information email: publishing@ygtmedia.co

ISBN trade paperback: 978-1-998754-29-8

eBook: 978-1-998754-30-4

To order additional copies of this book: publishing@ygtmedia.co

FROM

HOT
Mess
to
Happiness

HEATHER LIND

CONTENTS

To my mom, who taught me to find the humor in life; my Auntie Heather, who taught me to be independent and enjoy all the adventures that life has to offer; and the love of my life, Norm Hermanns, who has always accepted me for exactly who I am and has my back no matter what.

INTRODUCTION

♡

MY ROCK BOTTOM

TRIGGER WARNING:
BODY DYSMORPHIA; EATING DISORDERS

I woke from my sleep into the warm glow of the mid-morning sun.

At first it felt nice, like the sun was welcoming me to a beautiful day full of possibilities. That lasted for about one second and then I felt the usual anxiety and sense of dread that had become a normal part of my life.

Another day about to start. A whole day of self-loathing, telling myself how worthless, useless, and fat I was. How could I face another day? How was I going to get through it? How would I avoid eating?

Suddenly I remembered the leftover Chinese food in the fridge and felt a jolt of happiness. The very thing I blamed for my gross, fat body was the same thing I loved more than life itself. It was my escape; it was my drug of choice.

Once I started thinking about it, I couldn't stop. The texture and savory flavor of the rice and noodles; the sweetness of the sweet-and-sour pork; the deep-fried chicken balls full of grease, sugar, and what felt like love. I was all alone. This was the perfect opportunity to lose control and enjoy food without anyone seeing. I had been "good" all week by only eating vegetables, so I felt justified in having that leftover Chinese food in the fridge. I felt excited—excited about the food and excited to be able to eat without feeling like I was being watched and judged. Now, I don't think anyone was actually judging me, but I felt extreme shame in my desire for food. Like wanting food was a sign of weakness and indulging in it was caused by a complete lack of self-control. I wanted people to think I was in total control and never did anything as shameful as stuff my face with food.

As I tore open the containers, I felt an almost desperate need to consume all the food. I dove in, shoveling the greasy, sweet, and savory food I would normally not allow myself to have into my mouth. I wanted this moment to never end. The first few bites were like heaven. The taste and texture soothed me and made me feel so happy.

After those first few bites, though, I couldn't even taste the food anymore. I was just shoveling it in. I thought that as long as I kept eating I'd keep feeling happy, even though bite by bite I started to feel more and more anxious, ashamed, and frustrated. I could feel the heaviness of the food in my stomach, and I hated feeling full. Thus, I was battling between wanting to keep eating so I would remain happy and wanting to stop eating because I was becoming physically uncomfortable. The food made my mental pain disappear momentarily, but it then caused the physical discomfort. And that physical discomfort led to more mental pain.

I kept eating. I wanted to stop but something in me was driving me to keep at it, as I wanted the happy feeling to last just a bit longer. Then the little voice in my head started telling me how out of control I was and how ashamed I should feel for what I was doing. It was that same voice that was always telling me how worthless, unlovable, stupid, fat, and ugly I was. It told me that there was no point to my life. I was a waste of space, and I didn't even have the ability to exercise a bit of self-control. It made sure that I never forgot how much of a failure I was.

I was disgusted with myself as I put away the now almost-empty containers. I hated myself and told myself that I was an out-of-control fat pig. I thought about purging but couldn't bring myself to do it. The thought of the food scratching up my throat and my face being splashed with toilet water made me want to just go back to bed, so I crawled in and sobbed. All I could think about was how stupid I'd been for eating all that food and how full my stomach felt. That full stomach was hard-core evidence that I had once again failed. I was a pig and always would be a pig. I just wanted to fall asleep so I could escape this reality.

This was not an isolated incident. Scenarios like this one had been happening to me for years . . . decades, actually. This time, however, instead of just feeling hatred toward myself, I felt hatred toward the lifestyle I was living, toward the eating disorder I had allowed to consume and define me. Sometimes eating disorders can seem glamorous and exciting. I used to love that rush I'd get from avoiding meals and finding new and exciting ways to purge. But this was the first time that I really felt hatred toward the eating disorder. I felt desperate. I just couldn't stand the idea of living every day hating myself and battling against my willpower. This was no way to live, and I didn't feel ready to die, even though there were many days I wished I would.

This was the beginning of the end. This was my turning point.

I was determined to go from hot mess to happiness.

The Power of Surrender

I desperately wanted to be happy, but happiness eluded me. *What's wrong with me? Why does life feel so hard? Why is it such an effort to just be? Why do other people seem so put together and I'm such a hot mess? Why is life so easy for everyone but me?* I desperately wanted to have what others seemed to have: happiness and an ability to live life without always second-guessing themselves, plus hating themselves and feeling like a failure.

But how do you go from hot mess to happiness?

I was looking for the following when I was struggling:

- Peace within myself.
- Something I could trust in.
- Guidance on how to eat healthfully rather than in a disordered way.
- A way out of always feeling anxious and depressed.
- To get myself together and live a functional life that didn't always feel like such a struggle.
- A way to stop obsessing about food and how my body looked.
- To be happy with myself and not feel "less than" just because my thighs were too big to fit in jeans.

I was stuck in the sad world I had created in my head. I had allowed a monster into my thoughts and that monster kept getting bigger and bigger until it became the ruler of my life. I settled into that sad world and assumed that I was destined to be there forever. But then one day the pain and frustration just got to be too much. I found my pain limit and suddenly I felt able to evict the monster! I was so desperate that I decided to surrender.

The word *surrender* can have negative connotations. Some people see surrendering as giving up. Surrendering is not giving up. For me, surrendering is accepting things for how they are and realizing that you have the power to change how you interpret things. You can work with your situation rather than fight it. Trying to control everything and panicking when things don't go just right is unhealthy and will keep you trapped in frustration and sadness. The only thing we can control is how we react to what's going on around us.

For me, surrendering meant taking control of my health. It meant that I was going to feed my body what it needed and stop punishing it for not being what I wanted it to be. The body I wanted was not even realistic—I was never going to be waif-like because I don't have the bone structure for it. It would have been like trying to change my height. What I do have is a strong body with lots of muscle, and once I accepted that as my reality, I was able to work with my body and not against it.

For me, surrendering meant **simplicity**.

Getting to a point where I was happy and really enjoying life was surprisingly simple. Please understand, however, that simple does not mean easy. Simple just means that the things you need to do are achievable. That's the great news! Getting healthy can be quite simple! You need to commit and put in the effort, but you don't need to over complicate things. Eating well and improving health and fitness is actually more achievable than you might think.

My hope is that my voice makes a difference for someone. You can hear the same message over and over again but it just doesn't sink in. Sometimes hearing that exact same message again, but from a different voice and in different words, is what it takes to make it really mean something. There have been many topics that I've studied that didn't quite land with me until I heard the exact same thing explained just a bit differently.

My goal is to reach people who are:

- struggling with body image
- sick of living a life where they dread waking up and have to face the world
- frustrated with being confused as to what "diet" will work

- sick of stupid diets that never result in long-term success
- tired of hating their life
- seeing others living a happy life and just want to do the same
- feeling bad about being depressed because of how it affects their loved ones and their professional life
- feeling like they just don't quite fit in

I've been working on myself for quite some time now, and life got messier before it got better. I would like to help you get through the so-called messiness easier and quicker than I did. First, I'll tell you about my own history so you have a better idea of where I'm coming from and can hopefully relate. I'll then give you some insights that worked for me on improving my mental and physical health. Finally, I'll provide some simple tips that you can implement to help you become a healthier and happier you. As I said, the key for me was to keep things simple. The simpler I made things, the happier I became. The happiness that I started feeling was my motivation to keep going.

This is what I want to give to you: a simple, realistic plan so you can really start to enjoy your life.

In this book, I talk about my journey from depression and ill health to finally learning who I really was and how to love that person and live a happy life. After discussing my early years and how they developed my mindset, I've split my story into two remaining sections, Mind and Body, and I talk about the most important lessons I've learned. My hope is that you can relate to the lessons and use them to help you with your own journey to health and happiness. The most important point to keep in mind is that a healthy mind and healthy body go hand in hand. I strongly believe that you can't have one without the other. We need to feed our mind with healthy thoughts and positive messages and feed our body with healthy, nutritious food. I also keep the lessons and the homework simple so they're not overwhelming. Take it one step at a time. Don't rush the process and don't be cruel to yourself if you don't always stay on track. Be patient and kind to yourself and enjoy this journey to a healthier and happier life.

IMPRINTS

In order for me to help guide you, it's important for you to get to know me. My own journey was centered mostly around body image and weight, but it's relatable to any situation where self-esteem is an issue.

THE EARLY YEARS

I got sick a lot as a child.

I was born with lung issues and was tested several times for Cystic Fibrosis. Around five years old, I caught a flu that landed me in the hospital because I was having problems breathing. I vividly remember the sterile smell of the hospital room, the chilly feel of the oxygen tent, and the isolating feeling of being so alone. I didn't know any other kids who were going through health issues, and I missed a lot of school. In fact, my teachers were concerned that I might be dying of something because I was absent so often.

I couldn't eat when I was sick, as I'd have no appetite. This caused me to lose quite a bit of weight. I loved all the attention I got from my mom (it made me feel extra special and extra loved), and she'd pretty much offer me any food I wanted to just get me to eat. My favorite food in the world back then was mashed potatoes and gravy. I can still taste them. I really did love that extra attention. I felt seen, and I rarely felt seen in normal day-to-day life.

When I'd get better, I'd regain the weight and life would go back to normal—Mom would no longer obsess over my lack of appetite, and my childish brain interpreted this as meaning that I wasn't special anymore. I just faded into the background. I believe this was the unintentional start of my yo-yo dieting that slowed down my metabolism.

I eventually learned that being sick made me special. All eyes were on me when I was sick. I deeply craved attention. I wasn't super good at anything, but being sick seemed to make people really care about me and provide me with a lot of extra attention. When you identify strongly with something at a young age, part of you is afraid to let go of it. You feel like you'll disappear or just become so uninteresting that no one will pay attention to you or love you. At an early age I identified as being the sick kid, and this persona of being an unhealthy person stayed with me well into adulthood. In hindsight, I believe that it was the biggest driving factor behind my eating disorder. I had a need to be sick so I would receive attention, and I knew at least one surefire way to be sick—I didn't eat.

I've struggled with weight most of my life. I was typically between ten and twenty pounds overweight, which isn't a lot, but it was enough to make people notice and say hurtful comments. From a very young age I had issues with my body image. I felt like I wasn't good enough because I was the chubby asthmatic kid who sucked at all sports. My self-esteem was very low.

My parents were constantly dieting and weren't shy about complaining about their own bodies. My mom always got so excited when she lost weight! One time we went on a family vacation to Newfoundland for a family reunion on my mom's side. She dieted so hard that she was the same weight as my older sister by the time we left for the trip. My mom said that she loved seeing all her family members, but she was most happy about being the smallest of her sisters. Thus, my interpretation of her behavior was that being fat was bad and that you needed to sacrifice and suffer to get rid of it so you could look good. And looking good equaled happiness.

My mom pointed out to me when I was eight that I was starting to put on too much fat. She told me that she and my dad were concerned about my weight gain. She explained that my dad had started gaining weight when he was around eight and got teased about it, and they didn't want me to suffer through the same experience. I now know that what my mom told me came from a place of love, but it was a lot for a sensitive eight-year-old to process. All I got from that talk was that there was something wrong with my body. I looked bad and, if I wasn't careful, people would start to make fun of me. What's an eight-year-old supposed to do with that kind of information? I didn't have control over the grocery shopping or cooking. I sucked at all sports, so I wasn't very active. How was I supposed to lose weight? I would soon learn.

I remember one day when friends of my parents came over for a visit. The man told my sister that she was getting taller; he told me that I was getting taller . . . and wider. I was crushed. When he left the room, my sister said he had been mean to me, but she was giggling when she said it, so it really didn't make me feel any better.

I also started to develop breasts around that age, so I got teased a lot. I was too young to deal with such body shaming. My friends made fun of my changing body, and my parents were worried that I was getting too heavy. The message I received was that my body was different and therefore not as good as everyone else's—it was unattractive. To me, that meant that I could never be loved because I looked so disgusting. Obviously, I was a really sensitive child.

It was around that time that my inner voice decided to focus on how "wrong" my body was: thighs too fat, stomach too fat, everything too fat. I wanted to look good in a bikini. Why would an eight-year-old even be concerned with looking good in a bikini? But I thought that if I looked good in a swimsuit, the boys would like me and pay attention to me. I thought that being skinny meant that you were good and acceptable. This was my thought process from a very early age, and that voice just got louder and louder until she was in complete control.

I also started my first diet before I was ten years old. I learned the calorie content of almost every food, and I found that restricting calories did result in my weight loss—Eureka! It made me feel like I was taking action to fix a problem, and I was so excited to be doing something that would make me a better person.

I started purging at fourteen. I was babysitting one night and had put the kids to bed before eating a huge bowl of popcorn. I felt so full and disgusted with myself once it was all gone. I then thought about how I had heard about girls making themselves throw up, and I figured that vomiting would be a great way to undo the damage I had done by eating way too much. I went into the bathroom and closed the door, as I didn't want to wake the kids. I stuck my fingers down my throat and made myself throw up the popcorn. I was so excited! I felt like I had complete control—I'd never be the fat one again! My boyfriend at the time knew what was going on and said he was okay with it as long as I was careful. I knew then that he also didn't want me to get fat, something that put more pressure on me to lose weight.

I was soon only eating the meals I had to, which were breakfast and dinner because my mom was a stay-at-home parent, but I'd try to purge them if I could get away with it. I gave away all my lunches at school and avoided situations where I'd be expected to eat. If I did find myself in a situation where I was expected to eat, I'd just say I'd already eaten.

Losing weight became an all-consuming obsession that ate away at me. Nothing mattered more than dropping pounds. I'd lose some and feel like I was on top of the world, then I'd inevitably gain it back and be completely devastated. For me, the problem with the elimination diet was that I'd eventually get so hungry that I'd end up bingeing on something and then not be able to purge because my mom was home, and she'd hear me. So, I'd drop some weight and then put it right back on plus a little bit more. I was slowly damaging my metabolism from a very young age.

In school, I was horrible at anything physically active and did anything and everything to get out of having to participate. I wasn't good at any of the sports they made us play, and I seemed to always let my team members down, something I felt a mixture of embarrassment and disgust about. I don't remember ever having any measurable amount of self-esteem. For me, I thought that punishing myself was the answer and that I deserved that punishment. I was too scared to stop punishing myself, because without punishment, who was I? Who would I become? How would I prove my worthiness? My motto became "the worse I feel, the better I am."

In high school, I started doing aerobics at the local recreation center. My classmate went to aerobic classes regularly and had invited me along. I felt so nervous going. I was used to making a fool of myself when trying to do organized physical activity. I was so surprised when I found that I LOVED it! I couldn't do the whole class without taking breaks, but no one made fun of me or got annoyed. Instead, the other ladies taking the class told me I was doing great and to keep it up. I felt accepted and welcomed by these women. I felt like I had found my place.

Unfortunately, aerobic exercise soon became an obsession, and I only did it to lose weight. I thought that if I ate as little as possible and moved as much as possible, I'd finally be thin and beautiful—my world would be perfect! That didn't happen. Instead, I'd lose weight quickly, put it back on just as quickly, and I'd spiral deeper into my depression as a result.

The obsession continued into teenagerhood. One memorable incident was when I was a teen working at A&W. It was my turn to go on my break and my supervisor told me to go ahead and put in my order. I told her I wasn't ordering anything, and she exclaimed, "You never eat the food here." This comment was made in front of one of our regular customers. He said, "Well she must eat a lot at home, then. Look at those hips." Once again, I was crushed and spent my thirty-minute break looking at myself in the mirror, telling myself how fat and gross I was.

For the next nearly twenty years I fluctuated between bulimia and anorexia but was never overly successful at either. I was so frustrated that I was never able to get skinny enough, and I was so angry at myself for not being successful enough to land myself in the hospital. Your thoughts get really messed up when you're in the grip of the disorder.

It's tricky to get out of that situation when you're not feeding yourself properly. The brain does not operate well when it's not getting nutrition. The hardest part of getting over an eating disorder is that when you're in it and your brain is not operating well, you can't see any benefit of getting healthy. You hate yourself too much to do anything kind for yourself.

The level of hatred I had for myself is indescribable. I took myself way too seriously. I put too much of my self-worth in the hands of the people around me. I felt like I was useless and ugly, and I hated my body so much. I believed that being kind to myself would be seen as a weakness, which is why you can't just tell someone who's stuck in it to "eat a sandwich" or "just stop purging" or "quit punishing yourself." In that state, punishing yourself is viewed as success.

Another facet of the eating disorder mindset for many suffering from it is the belief that you have to be perfect. If you're perfect, everyone will love you. If you're perfect looking, everyone will think you have it all together. They'll think you're strong and in charge of your life. You are in control! But the reality is the total opposite. When you're in it, you're a mess! You can't concentrate. You can't give your best to the people around you. You know deep down that you're failing at life and having that knowledge makes you want to punish yourself even more. I felt like I deserved to be punished. I think I wanted to be punished—I craved it. If I was feeling bad, it distracted me from worrying about what people thought about me, something I think made me feel more powerful too. My superpower was to be able to get through each day even though I was feeling so bad and that it took absolutely everything for me to function. It made me feel more successful in that I was able to do all the tasks I needed to do even though it was a huge struggle.

Somewhere in my life I had decided that struggling was the mark of true success. My self-loathing went on for almost thirty years, as I navigated several different career paths.

I THINK I'LL BE A SCIENTIST!

When I was in high school and started thinking about my future, I planned it all out: attend college or university, get awesome grades, graduate, get a job in my chosen field, then live happily ever after.

My first career choice was biotechnology. I chose this field for two main reasons. First, I wanted to impress people. I had an interest in science so wanted to specialize in something scientific and thought that saying "I'm taking biotechnology" would impress others.

Second, I was able to take the course at a school that did not require four years of high school French. I did not enjoy French class. The British Columbia Institute of Technology had a great program that was only two years long. I was in a rush to get my life together, so this seemed like the perfect amount of time to get my education done. It was an intense course, and I didn't get the same kind of grades that I had earned in high school. But I did get through it, and after a lot of persistence, I was hired at the lab where I had done my work experience.

I did it! I was set for life! Smooth sailing here on in!

As it turns out, those were not very good reasons to choose a career path, something that became painfully obvious during the three years that I worked as a lab tech. My working at the lab seemed like a good, stable choice. My parents were proud of me, and when I told people what I did for a living, they seemed impressed, which is what I wanted. I liked telling people what I did—I worked in the first DNA identity testing lab in Canada—but that was about the only joy I got out of it. I was shocked and dismayed when I came to realize that I hated my job and that it was sucking the life out of me.

And I really did hate it. The theory behind what I was doing was very interesting, but I found being a lab tech to be mind-numbingly boring. As a lab tech, I felt like I was always trying to be a person I wasn't. It felt wrong, and little by little, it made me feel miserable about my life. I loved the people I worked with, but every day was the same thing over and over again.

My depression and anxiety got worse. I called in sick often and started feeling like I couldn't leave the house. My life looked good on paper, but I was miserable. I was so frustrated because I couldn't understand why I was so miserable even though I'd done everything right. I had what I set out to get. It was supposed to make me happy. The problem was that instead of trying to figure out what I wanted to do with my life, I tried to figure out what others wanted me to do with it. What a huge letdown.

And so, I came to the crushing conclusion that being a lab tech was not my path. But now what? I'd used student loans to go to school. There was no money to go back to school, and I sure didn't want to get myself into even more debt. What the hell had I done? I'd wasted all that time! I was in a really bad place mentally.

I decided to quit my job at the lab and move to a new community. I moved in with my sister and looked for work in my field even though I hated being a lab technician. When I couldn't find something, I took on a few different jobs. I worked at a couple of restaurants, and in retail for a bit. And at first it was okay. The huge pressure of trying to do well in a career that I hated was gone. Unfortunately, I got very bored and felt disappointed in myself. This was not supposed to be how things turned out for me. I was supposed to become a great scientist.

While I was living in this new community, I met who was to become the greatest love of my life. He saw all sides of me. It wasn't easy for me to let someone see everything, as I really didn't want him to leave me, and I was afraid that if he saw the real me, he would definitely run away. I wanted to be the perfect girlfriend even though there was absolutely no pressure from him for me to be perfect. He assured me that he loved me no matter what. I slowly let down my guard to test the waters. He saw some ugly stuff and he didn't leave. I didn't have to do anything to impress him or to keep him. I could just be me.

I think this is where I did most of my growing. I was in a situation where I could be me, and that was enough. The pressure to be a certain way lifted, and I started to learn who I really was and that who I was, was fine. I started to develop a sense of humor about myself rather than being overly critical. Life started being more fun and more interesting.

In my head I had thought my life had to go a certain way: graduate high school, go to college or university, get a job in the field I studied for, then live happily ever after. I was in such a rush to get everything lined up the way I thought it should be that I didn't take the time to discover what I actually liked doing. Science was interesting, but in looking back, I realize that my happy place was being at the gym. I found myself thinking more about the gym and when I could leave work to go to the gym. It never occurred to me that I could make a career out of it. I was in such a rush to get everything put together neatly in the correct box that I forgot to check in with myself. I was more concerned with what looked good, with what I thought would impress people, that I totally lost myself. It had never occurred to me to take time to discover myself and what made me happy.

I was in love with the gym—it's where I felt like my true self: sweaty and unstoppable.

Luckily, my boyfriend was open to a more nontraditional route to success and happiness, and he encouraged me to quit the safe, stable job that was making me miserable so I could study fitness and become a personal trainer and group fitness instructor. He let me discover what made me happy. There was no pressure to impress anyone or do what was expected of me by others. I was finally free.

Sometimes you need to take a leap into your biggest fear in order to fix what's not working for you. Everything in you might be telling you not to do it, but sometimes you must do the hard things that you've been fighting against in order to live a life that feels worth living.

So, I embarked on my next career choice: Personal Trainer!

I Think I'll Be a Personal Trainer!

I really jumped into consistent physical activity in my twenties. I loved going to aerobic classes. I loved the weight room. It was good that I now had physical activity that I enjoyed, but of course I took it too far by working out twice a day. In fact, one day I was called into a meeting at the YWCA, the gym where I worked out and volunteered. It was an intervention, and not for alcohol or drug use; they were worried that I was over-doing it.

While I was overindulging in my drug of choice, I was also doing my best to consume as little food as possible. The word fat had such negative connotations for me that I'd started to fear all fat and tried to eliminate as much of it as possible from my diet. I replaced fat with sugar-filled, low-fat or non-fat foods and all the diet pop I could drink, and I smoked cigarettes to combat my hunger. These bad habits did nothing to improve my appearance, but I continued to fight my weight and became increasingly unhealthy and irritated. The YWCA was right to intervene. I thought that the more I worked out, the skinnier I'd get, and all I wanted was to be skinny.

I was happy I had made the career change from lab technician to personal trainer, but I was more motivated by the possibility of weight loss for myself than for my clients. I thought being a trainer would magically make me fit. I figured if I placed myself in that position, I'd force myself to have the willpower to lose the weight because I'd have the pressure of people watching me.

Well, they watched me all right. I'd lose weight and get compliments, then I'd gain weight and get comments about how big I was getting. One day my boss at a gym where I worked at the time took me aside and said I should try to lose fifteen pounds so I'd represent his gym better. In his defense, he was discreet about it and said it as nicely as possible. At that same gym, however, a not-so-discreet fitness instructor told me that it's very important to look a certain way and that a chubby personal trainer who's out of shape would not attract clients or be taken seriously. I was devastated.

I was a personal trainer who smoked cigarettes, consumed as much diet pop as possible, and ate as little as possible. I still had poor body image and low self-esteem. Because I smoked, drank, and binged and purged, I felt like an impostor. On my days off, I'd start my morning with vodka in my coffee or whiskey in my tea. I certainly wasn't a picture of good health and was definitely not in a position to tell others how to take care of themselves. Here I was, portraying myself as a person who was healthy and could help others get healthy, when behind the scenes, I was leading an unhealthy life.

On occasions when I'd be out with friends and enjoying a cigarette, I'd always be looking over my shoulder to see whether any of my colleagues were around. Additionally, I'd visit clients after a night of heavy drinking, probably stinking of booze. I was helping people learn more about proper nutrition when I was doing my best to starve myself. It was a weird place to be—it was unauthentic, and it weighed heavily on my conscience.

I felt like I was in the right industry for me, however, so I cleaned up my bad habits to the point where I stopped feeling like a hypocrite. I had my "safe foods," including non-starchy vegetables, diet pop, and all the coffee and sugar twin I wanted, but I knew they were not enough to nourish me and make my life livable. So, I started eating oatmeal with protein powder for break-fast. For lunch I'd have a salad, but instead of just having lettuce and whatever light or non-fat dressing I had on hand, I'd add lean protein like skinless chicken breast and make my own salad dressing. I only used vinegar for dressing at first. Adding oil was too much to even think about, so I didn't force myself. Dinner was similar to lunch.

I was cautious in the beginning. I avoided certain foods like bread, pasta, and anything that was fatty. I knew that if I pushed myself too hard and if I saw too much weight gain, I'd give up. I had to do it slowly and at my own pace and add foods that I felt okay about but still had enough nutrition to be healthy.

My ultimate goal, though, was to repair my relationship with food and with myself.

TAKING STEPS TO CLEAN UP THE HOT MESS

When I was deep into my eating disorder, I was truly vicious to myself. I would physically punch my own stomach and tell myself that I was a fat, useless pig. Part of this behavior stemmed from a deep hatred I had built up for myself, and part of it stemmed from the fact that I was malnourished. My brain just wasn't functioning properly. To get out of that cycle was very difficult. It was when I finally hit my rock bottom that I decided to surrender to what I had learned about proper nutrition and apply it to myself.

I am so grateful that I had an interest in nutrition, as it is what led me to taking an amazing nutrition course. The course explained how nutrition worked and how our cells are affected by what we eat. It made sense even though in the back of my mind I was thinking that it would never work for me because I was somehow different from "normal" people. Every fiber of my being was convinced that there was no way proper nutrition was going to change me. To me, proper nutrition meant getting fat. It also meant caring for myself and loving myself, and I saw no reason for that. I felt like I didn't deserve to be loved or cared for. When you're in the eating disorder mindset, it feels impossible to do the things that you need to do to be healthy and happy. You feel like you're the one exception to the rule. You know that proper nutrition makes sense for others, but you don't trust your body to do what everyone else's seems capable of accomplishing. Also, taking care of yourself is not at all a priority. If anything, you want to punish yourself more and remind yourself how awful you are. It's a very sadistic disorder.

Thankfully, I decided to take a chance, to surrender and try doing what I learned from the course. I jumped in even though I was scared, promising myself that I'd give it a chance. I'm a very determined person. My mom used to call me stubborn! As it turns out, stubborn is an awesome way to be!

There was a lot of wavering in the early days of getting healthy. My metabolism was damaged. My body wanted to store as much fuel as possible in case I started starving it again. Putting my trust into the science behind proper nutrition and be okay with how it played out was probably the hardest thing I've ever done. I was handing over control to something outside of myself.

My biggest accomplishment was surrendering to the idea of feeding myself healthy food and not getting angry with myself for eating. I did put on some weight as my body became healthier, but I didn't get fat—I got healthy. Sounds good, right? But it was scary. I knew that if I saw numbers "proving" I was still a fat, useless pig, I'd give up. Fortunately, I'd had enough of the bullshit and threw out my scale and measuring tapes.

Once I got my nutrition under control, my mental state changed completely. I was lucky because I was stubborn enough to stick with the new plan long enough for my brain to start functioning better. I was actually able to feel more positive about life and my abilities. I got stronger, and as the depression and anxiety started to lift, I was able to use that fuel to keep at it.

Making necessary changes was easier than I expected, but it was a struggle at first because I had to be okay with some temporary weight gain and had to stop obsessing about how I looked. One trick I used was avoiding mirrors (or at least limiting the time I spent looking at myself). I also set the mirror at an angle so I could only see my body and not my face. Somehow that helped me look at my body objectively; I was able to look at my body as if it belonged to someone else. I mean, if I saw a person with the same proportions, I wouldn't consider them fat. Another trick I used was to look at myself, but not for too long. I'd look for something I liked and then quickly walk away because I knew the longer I looked, the more things I'd find wrong.

I had to fight the mean girl in my head every single day. I also had to be kind to myself and in the beginning of my transformation, that felt very wrong. The key is to know what will trigger you and then do your best to eliminate the triggers. But a warning: you can't eliminate them all. For instance, you don't ever want to tell a person fighting an eating disorder that they're looking healthy. To me, "you're looking healthy" was that person's polite way of telling me I was looking fat. That casual comment often set me back a few steps, and I'd go back to restricting calories and using various purging methods. To this day I hate it when someone tells me

I look healthy. It feels like a backhanded compliment.

People who want to help their loved ones get past an eating disorder need to understand that the person's mind is not working normally due to malnutrition. Advice like "just eat" or "just stop purging" or "do this for yourself" doesn't work. We're not stupid, we're just stuck in a really horrible mindset. I felt so guilty for causing my loved ones' grief, and that guilt fueled my self-hatred and my eating disorder. It's tricky: malnutrition affects your brain, and your affected brain keeps you from nourishing yourself to a healthier state. (For facts about eating disorders, please visit the Resources section at the end of this book.)

I had to fight to keep moving forward on my journey to good health. I didn't always win the battle, and that's where having patience and kindness toward yourself comes in. I still revisit my eating disorder sometimes, but it's only for brief periods and I am able to pull myself out of it.

Something that really helped me stay on track was noticing the energy I had. This energy allowed me to participate more in life and enjoy it. There are numerous people out there in the world who have never actually felt what it means to be healthy. They're not taking proper care of their health and assume feeling like crap is just a normal thing, especially as they begin to age.

It's not normal! If you have constant aches and pains but no injuries, that isn't normal! I know young people who move like they're way older, and I know people in their sixties, seventies, and even eighties and nineties who move with ease and enjoy an active life. Good nutrition and consistent appropriate exercise are your keys to being healthy and mobile.

It took some time, but as I started feeding myself properly, my mind started to change. It was like coming out of a really thick fog. I could see that the way I was treating myself would never get me what I wanted out of life. And I started enjoying my life. It was quite the turnaround for me, and to this day I know I will never go back to who I was when I was deep within my eating disorder, as I can still remember how anxious and depressed I felt. I'd wake up in the morning with a feeling of panic, which would then turn to a feeling of dread. Some days my anxiety was so bad that it led me to call in sick for work because I felt like I couldn't leave my apartment. However, when I stopped the war between me and myself, it opened me up to the simple pleasures of life. It let me discover what I was good at and pursue it, even though it wasn't a traditional route.

I THINK I'LL START A BUSINESS!

In 2012, feeling better than ever, I opened a small fitness studio. I was so excited! This was my dream! It was hard work, but thanks to the support of my boyfriend and help from so many great people, I did it!

Everything was wonderful until I realized that I wasn't going to be able to keep it running. I started my business with a loan from the bank, and I paid it all off. One of my proudest days was when I made that final payment on my loan. The problem was that I had only asked for what was probably about half of what I actually needed. At the time, I had absolutely no idea what I was doing. When I needed more money, I used my credit cards, and that got out of hand fast!

In 2018 I realized that I could no longer afford rent, and my debt was ridiculous. I'd made it six years, but the rent kept increasing and I was not very good at running a business. I'm an awesome fitness instructor and personal trainer, but running a business is not my thing. My accountant told me that I was not a "numbers girl" when it came time to file my taxes after the first year. He made me promise to never do my own books again.

A very generous and caring man who was a regular at my studio gave me a loan without asking me if I wanted it because he knew I'd say no. After he left that day, I cried out of relief and happiness. I slowly paid him back, another proud achievement in my life. The last thing I wanted to do was let him down. There are some really special people in the world, and I was lucky to have had so many in my life. But even with the extra help, I was drowning. I felt deep despair and embarrassment that I wasn't going to be able to make ends meet. It had never occurred to me that I could fail at growing this business, so it was difficult for me to acknowledge that fact. I put all I had into that studio, but it still wasn't enough. My skill set was not in building a business, so in the end, I had to accept that and let go of my studio.

I could have curled up in a ball and felt sorry for myself, which is what I really wanted to do, but I didn't. I let myself mourn the loss of my studio for a while, then finally asked myself, "What is the lesson here? What is the freaking lesson I'm supposed to learn?"

I searched for the lesson. It wasn't hard to find.

I am not cut out to run a business. When I thought about it, I'd only started my business so I could teach as many classes as I wanted and do them my way. Apparently, however, if you're going to start a business, you should have a plan for growing that business. My strength is being a personal trainer and fitness instructor, and I realized that I don't need my own studio to do the things I love and am most passionate about.

Ideally, business owners should work on their business, not in their business. And all I wanted was to work in my business—this realization was my lightbulb moment. I didn't need all the pressure of trying to grow a business. I wasn't thrilled about losing it, but I did eventually feel appreciation for the lessons I learned. I now knew what not to do! I should have done much more research before jumping in like I did, but going through that whole experience forced me to grow as a person and learn to accept that not every idea is a good one. Plus, I learned that if things don't work out, my world will not blow up.

I think the best lesson I learned from this experience, however, is that sometimes what you need isn't exactly how you picture it. I learned that if I feel like I'm having to fight every step of the way, it's probably a good sign that I'm not doing what's right for me. It's 100 percent okay to try something out and then change your mind if it doesn't feel like the right fit. It's all part of the adventure!

I'm still running my own business as a personal trainer and group fitness instructor, but I'm doing it in a way that fits my life and temperament a lot better.

CHOOSING HEALTH AND HAPPINESS

It took some time, but I eventually got to a healthy point where I am now taking care of myself and am able to serve my clients properly.

Here's what helped me get healthy and stay healthy:

- Giving in and trusting the science of proper nutrition.
- Paying attention to my mood changes and feeling optimistic about life.
- Letting the mean girl in my head run her mouth without reacting to her.
- Taking great joy in feeling healthy.
- Reminding myself that I am strong both mentally and physically and can stay that way.
- Not beating myself up if I happen to indulge in past unhealthy behaviors now and then.

The eating disorder lifestyle is very seductive. To this day when I'm feeling down about myself, thinking about starting it again and how I'd hide it from everyone still gets me excited. Thankfully, that excitement fades as I think about all the facets of it and how it destroyed me before and could very well again. It was a dark place, and I know I never want to go back there again. I still have days where I'm hard on myself and the dark thoughts come again, but I remind myself how bad it was to live that way and pull myself out of it. And I got to this point by reaching my rock bottom. But as it's said, the great thing about rock bottom is that you can only go up from there. How's that for reframing how you think about things?

MIND ♥

♡

MAKING FRIENDS WITH YOURSELF

Most of us are told that we should love and accept ourselves, but what happens when you just can't? What happens when you hate yourself and you feel like life is daily torture? What happens when you interpret your experiences as proof that you just aren't good enough?

I often felt guilty for indulging in depression and anxiety, as I had nothing in my outside life that was making me suffer. All my suffering was self-inflicted. My childhood was great, for the most part, and I had everything I needed. I felt that I didn't deserve to feel so bad when nothing awful had happened to me. So many people struggle with such challenging lives, and there I was, feeling sorry for myself for no reason. I was the one creating problems for myself.

Maybe it was because both my parents were depressed? There have been studies that show a possible genetic predisposition to depression when a parent suffers from it (please visit the Resources section for more information). My parents didn't talk about their mental health, but I think kids, especially overly sensitive ones, pick up on it. Maybe my depression stemmed from my low-quality diet? Maybe I thought life was supposed to be a struggle and since I didn't have any major struggles, I felt compelled to create my own?

All I know for sure is that I got to a point where I just couldn't stand living that way anymore. I wanted to be happy and enjoy life, and I didn't want my happiness to be dependent on how much weight I gained or lost. I'd had enough of feeling sorry for myself.

Minds are powerful, and what you believe about yourself will become your reality. That may sound like bad news, but it's actually great! Why is this great news? Because you have the power to change everything you believe to be true about yourself! Even if life seems bleak right now, you can take comfort in the fact that you can change. I did. I used to be stuck in a mindset that kept telling me how worthless I was and how pointless my life was. I was obsessed with finding the negativity in everything. I dreaded waking up in the morning. I dreaded being out in public where people could see how imperfect I was. I dreaded life with every fiber of my being. And believe me, changing my thinking, and therefore my life, was not at all easy. It wasn't a straight line from there to here. It was work, and I faced a lot of failures along the way.

Here's the thing, though. It was totally worth it.

When I finally got to a healthy place, both mentally and physically, I could not believe how amazing I felt and how much time I'd wasted being in that depressed state. I was actually excited about life, and there were many parts of my life that brought me extreme pleasure. Life wasn't all about me and that nagging voice in my head telling me that I was too fat. My life finally felt like it had purpose. I finally made friends with myself.

It took me a long time because I was fumbling through it all on my own. But I'm here to help you. Do you want relief from the pain you're feeling? Do you want to feel like you're a productive member of society who deserves a good life? You can make changes, and I can help shine the way.

In order to become happy with yourself and feel joy in life, you first need to get to know who you are, accept who you are, and even celebrate who you are. And believe me, we really do need to celebrate ourselves more! Let's talk about some tools that you can use to help you do just that!

The Mean Girl in Your Head
TRIGGER WARNING: SELF-ABUSE

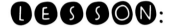

LESSON:

Self-acceptance takes practice and patience.

Anyone who has ever been teased or bullied knows all about mean girls (or boys). We do our best to avoid them, but did you know that most of us allow a mean girl (or boy) to live rent-free in our head where they make us feel like we're not as good as everyone else? Maybe your inner voice is loud and relentless, or maybe it's a bit quieter, but it's always there in the background, thriving on your misery. Whatever type of inner mean girl/boy lives in your head, you need to learn how to quiet them or, better yet, kick their ass to the curb!

I used to have a very close relationship with that voice in my head. I remember having it at an early age. It was always picking apart everything I did and finding what was wrong with it. It would find the negative side of everything. Even if I did well at something, that voice would tell me that it still wasn't as good as what other people did.

Things my inner mean girl said:

- You're a fat piece of shit.
- You suck at everything.

- Your sister is the pretty and smart one, and you got nothing. Better work hard to at least be the skinniest so that you have some sort of redeeming quality.

- No man will ever love you, and if they act like they do, there's some sort of ulterior motive because you've got nothing good to offer. Better lose more weight to keep him interested.

- The worse you feel, the better you are.

- If you starve yourself, you can at least be the skinniest one, but you're not even good at something that simple.

- Let's take the day off work and just eat everything!

- I can't believe you did that you fat, useless bitch—better go purge.

- You didn't do a good enough job of purging, and now that food that's left in you will turn to fat and everyone will see what a failure you are.

- Let's get drunk.

Why is it so hard to accept ourselves for who we are? Why are we so hard on ourselves? Why do we question ourselves? Why can we see beauty in others but pick ourselves apart? Why is it we can have so much love for others and absolutely none for ourselves?

Given the chance, the mean girl will take over and not shut up. But practice ignoring her, and she'll slowly disappear. She'll probably always be lurking in the background, but you have the choice not to listen to her. I liken it to a child having a tantrum and letting them do their thing until they get bored because they're not getting the reaction they want. I found that for me, if I let the terrible thoughts exist without getting involved, they went away and the mean girl got a bit weaker each time.

Try this exercise: Listen to what you're telling yourself in your head. Better yet, write down exactly what you're telling yourself. Next, ask yourself whether you would ever say those comments to your best friend. The answer, for me, was hell no! What I was telling myself about myself was far too cruel to ever say to anyone else. Take a second to really think about it. It's a bit mind blowing for anyone who is used to being super critical of themselves.

Here's what you can do, starting today, to be more self-accepting and kinder to yourself:

Stop spending time picking yourself apart in the mirror. Take a quick look, focus on the positive, then walk away because you know that if you spend a second longer you will find something you hate. Always leave on a high note!

If you do succumb and find something negative about how you look, make yourself find two positive things about yourself. These can be anything. Maybe your hair turned out great today, maybe you like how wonderful your outfit looks, maybe you like your makeup, maybe you were super productive today and got a lot of work done. It can be anything—just be sure that for each negative comment you give yourself, you make yourself find two positives.

List out all your positive attributes. My list was small to start and yours might be too. It might only be one thing. Keep adding to that list.

Do activities that make you forget about time. Have you ever been doing something you love and then you check the time and can't believe that an hour (or hours) has passed without you even being aware of it? Do that activity more often! For example, I love music. As a spin instructor, I like to pick a playlist and then design my ride around the music. I get so into it that I'm not aware of the passing of time. I'm completely lost in the music, and it brings me a huge amount of joy. I also love jigsaw puzzles. This might not seem like the most exciting way to spend time, but doing them relaxes me and I'm not stressing out about anything. Find your bliss. It doesn't even need to be anything productive. If you love Candy Crush, schedule a time in your day where you can crush candies and not worry about anything else. Think of it as a mini-holiday. A break from reality.

If you're feeling down, write out what you'd tell your best friend if they were feeling what you're feeling. Read those words back to yourself anytime you start feeling down. Learn to give yourself the love that you would give to your best friend.

Allow yourself to enjoy "me" time. Watch the "so bad it's good" TV show. Do something artistic and creative. Walk around your house naked while singing at the top of your lungs. Dance to your favorite music. Use your alone time to enjoy yourself in any way you want. You may even start looking forward to that time alone with yourself.

Allow yourself to be unapologetically you! Don't think about what others might be thinking about you, because you have no idea what they're thinking or why they're thinking it. Enjoy you and all your unique qualities.

To be truly happy, you need to be friends with yourself. You can never escape yourself, so the only option is to accept and love yourself by being as kind and patient with yourself as you would with your best friend. Once I latched on to this mindset, everything started to fall into place. Give yourself time, though. This can be a tough exercise at first, but I promise that you'll never regret becoming friends with yourself.

Here's what you're "supposed" to do:
Accept yourself for who you are and treat yourself
how you'd treat anyone else you love.

Here's what I did:
For most of my life I fought myself.
I hated myself and punished myself
for not being good enough.

How that worked out for me:
Badly. It makes me sad when I think of all the years
I wasted being miserable when I should have been
enjoying who I was and the body I was in.

What are you going to do?

Write It Down

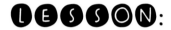**:**

Writing down your thoughts helps you process your feelings without having to worry about being judged. Be grateful for everything, even the seemingly small things.

Journaling. I came to this practice relatively recently and was surprised by how much it helped me.

While I was entrenched in my eating disorder, my brain didn't have the nutrients it needed to see clearly and notice small things that were so positive. As my nutrition improved and my brain recovered, I slowly began seeing improvements in my mental state. I started taking pleasure in smaller things like hitting all the green lights on my way to work. My world became brighter, and I began paying attention to all the positivity in life. I started to feel gratitude.

The next step was recording the things I was grateful for. When I first heard about writing out a gratitude list every day, I thought the idea was stupid. That whole "let the universe know how grateful you are and it will provide you with everything you need" made me roll my eyes. But then one day I did it. I'm not sure what sparked me to try it, but one morning it just felt right.

I made a list of ten things I was grateful for and then journaled every single morning after. Most days had the same list with maybe one or two new things, but I always listed ten things. I was amazed how doing this made me feel. It started my day on a high note.

More and more I started thinking about all I had to be grateful for, and there were a lot of things. I felt a sense of lightness, like the fog I had been living in was finally lifting. I even got to a point where I couldn't even imagine being the sad person I once was. Journaling made me really think about all the great aspects of my life: my very short commute to work, my quiet morning time to myself, my amazing cats, etc. These simple things gave me so much pleasure and comfort and all I had to do was pay attention.

I now regularly journal early in the morning. I'm the only one up, it's quiet outside, and I'm able to focus on the thoughts I'm having. In addition to writing out my gratitude list, I also include my to-do list for that day. And when I'm feeling really stressed, I write down all the things I'm thinking in my notebooks. Let's face it—at some point most of us have thoughts that we think might sound a bit bonkers to the outside world. Logically, you know they sound weird, but they're in your head and you need to get them out, which is part of the healing process. Some people hugely benefit from therapy, but even just writing your thoughts in a private notebook is quite healing.

There's something very powerful about bringing pen to paper and writing down your thoughts. It's a great way to process what's happening. It's an opportunity to get those loud, cluttering thoughts out without having to find a person who is willing to listen and won't judge. I never reread my notes, and I always throw out the journal when it's full. That way, I set my thoughts free.

If you would like to try journaling but aren't sure how, here's how to start: Write a list of five things you are grateful for. Do it every morning before you head out to face your day. Notice how much lighter you feel when you've given some attention to those small things that make life so great.

★

Here's what you're "supposed" to do:
Give those thoughts that you'd rather not talk to
someone about a bit of life by letting them live on a
piece of paper so you can process what's going on.
Practice gratitude daily.

★

Here's what I did: I got a late start,
but I gave my "unspeakable" thoughts a chance
to live for a tiny bit of time in my private notebooks.
I practiced gratitude daily.

★

How that worked out for me: Amazingly well.
Instead of churning those thoughts around in my
head, I set them free by acknowledging them and
writing them down. This allowed my brain to process
what was happening, and once processed, it was
easier to let them go. I felt better about life and
became a very happy person.

★

What are you going to do?

No One Is Alone

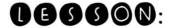 **:**

When struggling, we often think we're alone, but if you take into account how many people there are in the world, it just makes sense that someone out there is going through something similar.

Feeling alone can be terrible. Humans are social by nature, and we need our support system. It used to be that isolation meant death. If you wanted to live, you needed a group of people for support and protection. Since the beginning of time, the people that flourished were the ones who stuck together and worked together to create something bigger than just themselves. There's strength in numbers, and we need to receive that strength and contribute to that strength.

That need for connection is deep within us all, even those of us who are a bit introverted. I love to have my alone time but too much of it drives me back to self-criticism, depression, and anxiousness. If you're stuck in your head, helping someone can bring some relief. A basic human need is to be helped and to help others. We need to be loved, and we need to love others. Share yourself with someone who needs support and help them with their struggles.

With the technology we have today, we can connect with people nearly anywhere in the world at nearly any hour. I may not always feel like being social or leaving my house, but I know that if I need a bit of feedback or some support I can connect through social media or send a private message to someone I miss. It is helpful to search for like-minded people in Facebook groups or on other social platforms. We are never alone and knowing that can be a great comfort.

A bit of a warning about social media, though. It can be great for you, or it can destroy you. It all depends on how you use it. Remember that people usually just post the great moments that happen when the lighting is perfect. Treat social media like a healthy nutrition plan. Consume the things that are good for you and give you energy and joy and cut out those that you know are going to make you feel bad. If you find yourself getting down on yourself after looking at social media, trim down who you follow to just people you know, love, and respect in real life who help you feel better about yourself.

On that note, another way to realize that you are not on your own is to reach out to family (either the family you were born into or the family you've created) and friends. I have a terrible habit of being lazy when it comes to friendships. I'm introverted and really do enjoy alone time almost to a fault. The problem, however, is that friends can sometimes interpret that as meaning I don't care about them or value them. If you tend to be like me, you might one day find out that your friends have moved on.

Stay in touch with the people you love and nurture them. In doing so, you'll most likely find that it will actually strengthen your own friendship with yourself.

Here's what you're "supposed" to do:
If you're feeling like you are alone in anything,
reach out to your support group.

Here's what I did:
I isolated myself a lot. I pushed friends away
and lost quite a few of those friends.

How that worked out for me:
Terribly. I felt more depressed and more anxious.
When I finally did start reaching out more for support, I felt so much better about life. I became less
self-critical. I even found that I was actually able to
help others find comfort. Nothing feels better than
knowing that you helped someone.

What are you going to do?

FINDING THE POSITIVE IN ANY SITUATION

Did you know that what you put out into the world comes back to you?

Maybe it sounds a bit flaky, but it's true: what you put out you get back. I've experienced this in many ways in my life, and I've seen others experience it as well.

Think about exercising, for example. There have been many times that I've started a workout or gotten ready to teach a class and all I could think about was how tired I felt. Then by the end of the workout, I was bubbling over with energy! Put the energy out and it comes back to you. And it doesn't just work with exercise and energy levels, it also works with how you view your world and how you show up in it.

I used to see the negative in everything. I'm a very sensitive person, which means I pick up on people's moods quite easily. I am aware of this habit now and just let it go, but as a kid I internalized it. When I began struggling with depression and anxiety, I thought it was all me. I thought that I was the one causing myself to be sad. I realize now that I was just really sensitive to what was going on around me and I internalized it all. It became normal to feel sad and see the negative in everything. Even in good situations I'd manage to find negatives. And when bad things happened to me, I'd think, *Of course that happened; life sucks and I suck.*

But somewhere along the way I started to notice the positives. My mom used to say that we have to find a way to laugh at life and ourselves. She said that life was too short to let little stuff get us down. Eventually, I took this advice to heart and started looking for the humor in life and focusing on good things, no matter how small or insignificant they seemed.

For example, I live in a tiny, expensive condo in Vancouver with my boyfriend. I could get caught up on the fact that we pay a lot of money for a little bit of space, but instead I think about how great it is to not have a lot to clean. I can vacuum the entire condo in about twenty minutes!

Another example of looking for positives is how I viewed the lockdowns and loss of work due to COVID-19. I could have spiraled into depression over the fact that my life had changed dramatically, and I had to almost completely reinvent myself. Instead, I looked at it as an amazing opportunity to write this book. The last lockdown also allowed me to be home with my cat, Ellen, for the last few weeks of her life. The positivity is there but sometimes you need to search a bit for it.

What's happening in your life right now? Can you find a way to see the positive (or maybe even the humor) in it?

In this next part we'll focus on how to let go of self-limiting thinking, how to find the lesson in the struggle, and how to stop spending too much time worrying about things we can't control. Your life is your opportunity to experience everything you want to so don't waste any time on thoughts that keep you tied down. We're all on this earth to experience our own journey; if you let it, it can be a very fun and interesting ride.

Live Your Life for You, Not for Others

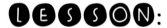

Let down your guard and be carefree so you can enjoy your life. Nobody cares as much as you think they do about what you're doing.

I've always been a bit envious of people who can do and say what they want even when it might make them look silly. I used to be an observer. If I was at a party and people were dancing, I'd watch. I desperately wanted to join them, but I was too afraid that I'd look like an idiot. But keeping my guard up kept me from participating in and enjoying so many things in life. For a while alcohol was my fix. In drunken moments I'd let myself have fun. Then I'd wake up the next morning and feel like all I'd done was look stupid.

A huge block between me and happiness and self-acceptance was trying to do what I thought I "should" be doing. I was always thinking about what other people thought of me and trying to figure out how to make them happy so they would accept me. I was looking for validation outside of myself. So nuts! I wanted the acceptance of others even though I didn't accept myself. Here's the thing: no one really expects anything from you. There is most likely no one obsessing over what you're doing, as they're too busy obsessing over what they're doing. When you think about it, it's ridiculous to believe that others are really spending that much time, or any time at all, thinking about what someone else is doing with their life.

Something that helped me feel free to be myself was taking group fitness classes. They were regulated, and I felt safe enjoying myself without worrying about what other people were thinking of me. And teaching fitness classes allowed me to let my true self shine through and have fun. I was in an environment where everyone was paying attention to me and listening to me because they wanted to. They wanted me to lead them. They were there to hear me and let me guide them. I felt safe to push my level of comfort into discomfort. I was able to joke with them and act like myself without fear of being ridiculed. I got positive reactions, and I felt on top of the world.

Still, sometimes people say things that hurt my feelings. When I'm bulking, I put on weight, some muscle and some fat. Occasionally, someone will feel the need to point out that I've gotten bigger. Comments like these used to crush me, and I'd be a mess for the rest of the day. I have to remind myself that they aren't attacking who I am, they are just making an observation. Then when I'm leaning out and getting close to stage time, I get lots of compliments on my physique. These comments used to make me unbelievably happy. A little too happy actually, so I remind myself that this, too, is just an observation from another person.

If someone makes a comment you don't like, whether about how you look or something you've done, remind yourself that it's just an observation from that person, and they are free to have their opinion. Just remember that their opinion doesn't matter as long as you're doing what you know feels right for you. Most people probably don't realize how hurtful their comment is to you, so don't let it get you down. When someone does comment on my body, I'm able to make a little joke about it and laugh at myself. It's such a freeing feeling to not care that much about how people are going to react to you. I just wish I could manage to do the same in all facets of my life.

When you put your energy into worrying about what others might be thinking about you, you rob yourself of a lot of joy. Can you imagine how great you would feel if you didn't spend time worrying about what others think? You absolutely don't have to worry! People are thinking about themselves way more than they're thinking about you or anyone else.

Let go of trying to live the life you think will be best for others and start living the life that is best for you!

★

Here's what you're "supposed" to do:
Live your life without fear of what
other people might think of you.

★

Here's what I did:
Aside from when I'm teaching classes,
I'm quite self-conscious and subdued in public.
The fear of possibly looking like an idiot
paralyzes me.

★

How that worked out for me:
Not great. I really do feel like I miss out on
a lot of fun by staying safe on the sidelines.

★

What are you going to do?

Fall in Love with the Process

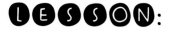:

You spend more time working toward a goal than you do enjoying the actual achievement, so if you want to be happy, you need to enjoy the process.

Have you ever felt like you're not getting anywhere? Like you're not where you should be? That you need to do more? I've heard this referred to as "striving but never arriving."

We often get so stuck on the outcome we're after that we forget to enjoy the process of getting there. And when you think about it, achieving the goal you set is just a second in time. The work to get there lasts much longer. If you don't enjoy the process of getting to your goal, you'll never feel fulfilled. There will always be something you're chasing.

Take fitness for example. If you set yourself the goal of losing some excess weight and only focus on the end result, you are going to become frustrated. Unfortunately, one workout and one day of eating well will not magically transform you into the strong, healthy person you want to be. It takes consistency. You need to be persistent and consistent. Thus, if you don't take time to find the joy in what you're doing, you'll get tired of it and give up before you reach your goal.

I know from personal experience how devastating it can be when I'm only focused on the outcome, and then when I reach that outcome, it's not as great as I thought it would be. This happened to me with my attempted career in biotech. I was so anxious to reach my goal of working in a lab that I didn't take the time to enjoy the process of getting there. Instead, I spent most of my time stressed out because I was so worried that I wouldn't reach my goal.

When I did finally achieve it, I was shocked by how disappointing it was. I had romanticized it in my head, but reality didn't even come close to how I'd imagined it would be. As a lab tech I felt like an impostor because I was doing something I hated. I was good at it, but I dreaded going to work. I'm grateful now that it happened that way, as that experience opened me up to taking a more nontraditional route to my career in fitness, which I love. In it, I've found my happiness in helping people get healthy, and I feel fulfilled and useful. I've found my passion and have finally started living.

The wonderful thing about life, once you open yourself up to it, is that you can experience as many passions as you like. Fitness was my first true passion. Since then, I've discovered other things that I'm passionate about and have tried out. Life becomes so much fun when you approach it with the same kind of openness a child does when approaching new opportunities and experiences.

Slow down. Enjoy the process. Make it a valuable part of your life. Approach your goals like road trips. Enjoy the scenery and take it all in. Keep in mind that your final destination may not be as great as you imagined. Be open to whatever unfolds.

★

Here's what you're "supposed" to do: Enjoy every step on your way to your goal. Don't let your joy and satisfaction be dependent on just reaching the goal itself.

★

Here's what I did: I was in the mindset that until I reached my goal, I was basically failing.

★

How that worked out for me: It stressed me out and most times when I achieved my goal I felt let down because I thought I'd be happier.

★

What are you going to do?

Learn to Be Present

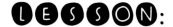:

**Worrying only causes stress.
The present is all we have. It's the only thing
that actually exists. Mind blown!**

I was such a stressed-out kid. I worried about EVERYTHING. I remember trying to fall asleep and being worried that the furnace was going to catch fire and burn down our house. I remember feeling stressed about things I had done wrong in the past and feeling like I was a bad person for having done them.

I was also scared of things for no real reason. When I would go to the fair with my family, for example, I wouldn't go on any rides because I was scared that something might happen. I hated going out fishing on my dad's boat because I was sure it was going to sink and we'd all drown. If there was something to worry about, I'd find it. If there was nothing to worry about, I'd search my brain until I was able to make something up to stress about. I have no idea why I was like that. My dad used to call me a worrywart, and he was right!

I carried that worry for everything with me well into my adult life. It wasn't until my early forties when I started reading Eckhart Tolle's work and learned that I was fighting a losing battle by stressing out about everything that I actually stopped worrying so much. When I stumbled across Eckhart Tolle, my inner world changed. (Visit the Resources section for more information on Eckhart Tolle.)

Worrying about things that have already happened is useless because there is absolutely no way to change them. For the most part, memories of the past are very inaccurate anyway. And being stressed about the future is also mostly futile because no matter how organized you are or how much you plan, you really have little control over the outcome. The future doesn't exist yet; all we can do is imagine it, and how we imagine it may not be how it occurs. COVID taught us that lesson over and over again. The only thing that actually exists is the present. The only real thing in your life is what is happening at this very second.

In hindsight, I realize that I spent way too much time imagining horrible outcomes to things I hadn't even tried to do. I used to live in the past and imagine how I'd live in the future. All that did was make me feel anxious and too afraid to try certain activities. I typically focused on negative past experiences; plus, I seemed to have an affinity toward imagining the worst for my future. No wonder I was so anxious.

I still catch myself ruminating once in a while. I'll imagine the worst case scenario for something and then question whether I should even try to achieve it. It sometimes feels like there are a few people living in my head! One always wants to focus on the negative side of everything, while another constantly tries to talk the negative one out of doing that. And then there's a third who has a perverse interest in what disaster is going to happen next, like you do when watching a particularly ridiculous reality show. Ever get the feeling that your life is a particularly ridiculous reality show?

Luckily, I catch myself having these thoughts and then push through anyway. If I wasn't able to push through, I never would have opened my studio, I never would have tried road riding, and I never would have tried competing in bodybuilding. At one point in my life I was in a mental place that made it hard for me to even leave my house. Overthinking the negative possibilities will leave you paralyzed. I would have missed out on some of the greatest experiences of my life if I had let my overthinking take over.

Living in the past or (what you think is) the future only results in stress. Our brain doesn't know the difference between actual events and imagined events. If you think about it, it makes you realize how careful you need to be with the thoughts you allow to exist in your head.

When I started to really understand this concept, so much pressure was lifted off me. I stopped feeling like if life didn't go as planned, then the world would come to an end or something even more horrific would happen. It also taught me to enjoy what's happening right now. It can be as simple as noticing how much I'm enjoying the feel of the couch I'm sitting on or as complex as enjoying every nuance experienced when engaging with another person without being distracted by negative thoughts in my head. Understanding this concept brought a higher quality to my life. I felt more at peace. I also picked up on many of the tiny things that people often miss in life: the simple things that bring about an immense amount of pleasure when you start noticing them.

All you have control over is making your plan, so do what you can do in the moment to work toward your goal and then see what happens.

What are you worrying about right now? What can you do right now that will help? It's perfectly normal to worry (worrying is one way we protect ourselves from danger), but you can't let worry take over your life. Take comfort in the fact that all you can do is what you can do in this very moment. The rest will come, and you'll do what you need to do when you need to do it. Stop overthinking, take a breath, and let go of thinking that you know exactly how things are going to work out.

The next time you're out for a walk, block out all your thoughts and just focus on what you're seeing, hearing, feeling, and smelling. I'm sure you've heard the advice to stop and smell the flowers. Try it! See the flower, touch it, smell it, and pay complete attention to it. If another thought enters your head, block it out. It's not important unless that thought is *Uh-oh! There's an angry-looking dog running right toward me!* Take the time to enjoy one thing at a time and completely immerse yourself in it, even if it's just for a few seconds. Keep practicing. It will become easier, and you'll become happier. Life takes on a richness that is so far beyond who and what you think you are. Life becomes pleasure.

All that really exists is the present moment. Enjoy your adventure.

★

Here's what you're "supposed" to do:
Stop worrying! Let go of the past and don't try to predict the future. Be present in every situation.

★

Here's what I did:
For most of my life I lived in a constant state of worry and regret. Once it was pointed out to me how much people tend to think about the past and future without noticing what's going on in the present, I started paying more attention to my thoughts and what was actually going on in the moment.

★

How that worked out for me:
I used to be anxious all the time and even had problems with leaving my house some days. After learning to be in the present, I felt happier, lighter, and more fulfilled with life in general.

★

What are you going to do?

Find the Lesson in the Struggle

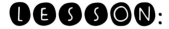

LESSON:

**You can't control what happens,
but you can control how you react.**

I like to try to find the lesson in everything.

"Change the way you look at things, and the things you look at change." I love this quote from self-help author Wayne Dyer (for more on Dyer, visit the Resources section).

One thing I've learned is that we absolutely cannot control certain outcomes. We also can't change what's already happened and we can't predict with one-hundred-percent certainty what will happen. What we do have complete control over is how we react to outcomes. How we frame them. We can see challenges as opportunities to learn and grow, or we can see challenges as the world hating us and wanting us to fail. One way will get you excited to learn the lesson; the other way will dim your light until there's nothing left.

You need to find the lesson in the struggle. I decided to believe that everything is interesting. Good, bad, or indifferent, there's a message and it's always interesting. The trick is to shut off the voice in your head that judges the situation. View things like a child would. When you watch young children play and explore, you can see that they don't have a judgmental bone in their body. They just take it all in with a sense of wonder. They learn about their world around them without labeling it. They take things as they come and just learn. It's unfortunate that we lose this ability as we get older. We become judgmental and cynical. Life becomes a lot less fun and interesting.

The good news is that life doesn't have to be this way. With some practice we can recapture the feeling of awe and wonder about the world around us. Think of life as a movie you're watching. Sometimes you might not like what you're seeing, but that scene ends and you get to watch what happens next. When I started having the attitude that everything is interesting, I felt like the pressure of the world lifted right off me. I began allowing myself to experience things, good or bad, and instead of reacting, I would try to look for what's interesting.

Now this doesn't mean that I don't get upset when things don't work out the way I want them to. I am human, after all. I let myself be upset, but I put a limit on the amount of time I let myself feel those negative emotions and then decide what I need to do to adapt and be happy again. In other words, I look for acceptance of the situation so I can move on.

Life is going to keep changing and most people don't like change at first because it's uncomfortable. But what are you going to do? Spend the rest of your days complaining? Some people do. Those people are very difficult to be around. Why would you want to live your life complaining about everything? Wouldn't it be better to figure out how to adapt and make the best of it? You may even discover that the change is better than how things were before it. You'll probably discover new opportunities that you hadn't considered. I wasn't thrilled when I had to close my studio, but it led me to finding work that allowed me to do what I love while also giving me a lot of free time to work on and discover other interests. If I had my studio today, I'm fairly certain I would not have had the time to write a book. Things change, we move on, and it's all very interesting.

I'd like you to take a moment here to think about something you struggled with in the past or something you're struggling with now. Do this somewhere quiet with no distractions and see if you can find the lesson in it. It may be difficult to find the lesson, especially if you're right in the middle of the struggle, but if you take the time to do this exercise, I think you'll find that you'll feel more optimistic and maybe even grateful for getting to experience the struggle.

By finding the lesson, you can find strength in the struggle. This will give you the confidence that you'll be able to handle anything that comes your way.

★

Here's what you're "supposed" to do:
Don't try to control what happens, and if things don't go as planned, DO NOT panic!

★

Here's what I did:
Tried to control everything and panicked a lot.

★

How that worked out for me:
Not good. I was a giant ball of stress from a very young age. When I finally accepted that I couldn't control everything and instead started to observe what was happening and just accept it, I became much more laid back.

What are you going to do?

DISCOVERING WHO YOU ARE

Have you ever asked yourself, "Who am I?"

Why do we feel the need to define in words who we are? Shouldn't we just know the answer intuitively? It can be very frustrating and almost impossible to figure out and, unfortunately, a lot of us think about who we are in terms of how we want others to think about us. We then get confused when we define ourselves by how we interpret the messages we receive and who we want people to think we are. I wanted people to think I was smart and had my life under control. I am smart but not in the way I wanted to be. I wanted to be the genius scientist that everyone respected and took seriously. I tried playing that part, but it was not the part for me.

Identifying with anything outside of yourself can be dangerous. It limits you and keeps you weighed down. It's like a ball and chain around your neck. We are constantly changing, which is a good thing. We need to evolve and keep growing! Evolution is how a species survives, and evolution means changing, but so many people get caught up in trying to be what they think their label is. If you decide to define yourself by one label, you could end up allowing fear to make all your decisions, which can stop you in your tracks before you even try new experiences. This has the potential to create limitations and anxiety.

When I gave up my lab tech job and started working toward becoming a fitness leader, I discovered that I felt a true passion for this new career path. I got excited thinking about what I'd be doing as a personal trainer. I started feeling really happy about it. Unfortunately, I had that mean girl in my head telling me it wasn't good enough. I wasn't going to impress people by telling them that I was just a personal trainer. Fortunately, I didn't let that voice stop me, and this is where letting go of a bit of control came in handy for me. Instead of deciding who and what I was, I started learning how to adapt to what was going on in my world. I questioned myself for taking this path, but I didn't stop working toward it. Something in me knew that being a personal trainer was more me than being a lab tech.

Stop asking yourself who you are and belittling the things you do really well. Tell that mean girl in your head to shut up so you can figure out what really makes you happy—what really brings joy into your life. When you know what brings you true joy, all you have to do is figure out how to share that with other people.

Life is about exploring new adventures, seeing how we react to these adventures, and letting ourselves exist without judgment. Everything is interesting when you take the time to look at it without labeling or judging it. Be like a child and learn from the things you experience without judging yourself or the situation. What's your passion? What comes so easy to you that you don't even really think about it? Maybe it's art. Maybe it's organizing things. Maybe it's caring for people and/or animals. Imagine being able to live in your joy while at the same time making a difference in someone's life. When you're working from a place of bliss, people will be drawn to you and your expertise.

Find your purpose. What's something that you've experienced? If you've lived through it, you're an expert on it, and someone needs your help. What might seem insignificant to you can be life changing for another who is suffering. Share your experiences so others can learn from your wisdom. There's no greater feeling than knowing that you made a positive impact on someone's life.

Do you know what your passion is in life? Do you feel like you have a certain purpose in this life? Maybe you're not sure. Or maybe you know what it is, but you feel like it's not that important. Or maybe you know what it is but you're afraid to pursue it because you're afraid to fail. In this next part we'll talk about finding your value and how to share what you have to give without trying to do it perfectly. You have more value than you probably realize and to not share that value would be a disservice to yourself and others.

Share Your Gold

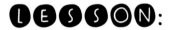:

We all have value, and we're all here to help one another. Don't act in a certain way just because you think it will impress people. Find something you enjoy and make a career out of it.

What things do you get fully immersed in? What's something that you do that makes you forget about time and anything else that's going on in your life? This is your passion, and you need to discover how to do more of it! Better yet, you should explore how you can make a career out of it so you can earn money while doing what you love.

Nearly everything I've done with my life so far has come with the nagging thought that I'm just not that good at it. I used to look for my faults, then get stuck on them. As I got older and wiser, I started to focus on my strengths. But my strengths weren't necessarily the things I wanted to be good at doing. I wanted to be a genius scientist and impress everyone with my amazing knowledge, but that didn't work out for me. Not even close.

As it turns out, I'm a really good group fitness instructor and personal trainer. I truly enjoy helping people, I love working out and listening to music, and I have a thorough understanding of how the body works and what it needs in order to keep working well. I'm most present in life when I'm teaching a fitness class or working with a client. This wasn't the impressive scientist career that I once thought I wanted, but it's something that I'm great at and can be fully immersed in.

So why didn't I become a personal trainer in the first place? In hindsight, I think it was because of how easy training people came to me, and for some reason I figured it couldn't be valuable if it was easy. I believed that I had to work myself to exhaustion in order to offer anything of value. What I didn't recognize at the time, however, was that what is easy to one person may not be easy to another. The person who finds it easy is meant to teach the one who struggles with it.

When you feel like something comes easy to you and therefore must not be of much value, take a second to really think about it. Think of two children, for instance. One can tie their shoes with no problem. It's super easy for them and they think nothing of it. The other cannot tie their shoes and thinks the other is a god because they can do this complicated task. We all have gold to share with others, even if we believe it's something insignificant. But no one is insignificant. We all have our talents.

On the other hand, if you feel like you're lacking knowledge in something, look for someone who has it. Don't be envious and think that you are less than because you don't have the same skill set. Be grateful because they can teach you what you want to learn. And if you're still not able to do it after they've taught you how, maybe you can hire them to do it for you.

When someone tells me I've made a difference in their life, I feel like I'm on top of the world. I used to wave off the compliment and think to myself that they were just being polite. Over the years I've learned that I really do help people and I am indescribably grateful for that gift.

Sometimes, even with all the positive feedback on my abilities as a trainer and group fitness instructor, I still feel like I should be better at it. Is this a bad thing? Maybe it's a good thing? I don't like doubting myself, but it does push me to always try harder, learn more, grow more. The lesson here is that if you feel like there's no room for improvement in something, maybe you've lost your passion for it.

With technology making the amazing advancements it has, there are so many options for careers. Maybe you're an influencer and you haven't realized it yet. Find what you love and start posting tips on Instagram. Become the expert people look to for advice. It may lead to writing a book or holding seminars and webinars on how to do that thing you love. There are endless possibilities, you just need to get a little creative.

We are all here to contribute to life—we can all chip in and make a difference. Everyone has strengths that can be shared with others, and it's our responsibility to learn as much as possible about those topics and skills so we can help others. So, figure out what you love doing; it's most likely something that comes easy for you. Don't second-guess your talent! Share the hell out of it.

Here's what you're "supposed" to do:
Love yourself, cherish your unique talents,
and share your gold with anyone who needs it.

Here's what I did:
Hated myself and tried to love myself
by making others happy.

How that worked out for me:
Not good. If I had known then what I know
now I would have started learning what
made me happy and how I could share that
with others much earlier than I did.

What are you going to do?

Scare Yourself

🅛🅔🅢🅢🅞🅝:

Life is growth. We need to let the growth happen and not limit ourselves because of stories we've been told. If you want to boost your self-confidence, do the things that scare you.

I wasn't always open to growth. There was a time when I had to have everything planned, and if something didn't go as I had planned it, it was devastating to me. I thought my life was meant to play out a certain way, and when it didn't lead to "happily ever after," I was miserable. I was raised to strive for security, to not take risks. Get a good job, save some money, and live well. It made life very stressful for me while I was trying to force this plan to work.

I've since learned that it's okay if things don't go as planned. Letting go of my career in biotechnology and pursuing my career in health and fitness was scary but exhilarating. In changing careers at such a young age, my mind was opened to the possibility that life doesn't always have to go as planned—and it doesn't always have to follow a conventional route. I realized that I had room to grow, that I could find myself and live a life that excited me. I learned so much about myself when I stepped out of my comfort zone and went for what my soul really needed, something that is largely in thanks to my boyfriend who encouraged me to chase after what makes me happy. I'm very fortunate to have him in my life.

Opening my studio taught me to be comfortable with a growth mindset. It taught me that what you have planned is not necessarily what's going to happen. It also taught me that the way things turn out is perfect even if it doesn't look exactly how I thought it would.

Taking part in photoshoots has also contributed to my growth mindset. I hate having my picture taken, so photoshoots make me very uncomfortable. The "old" me would have never even considered hiring a professional for a photoshoot! The mean girl in my head would have told me that I didn't look perfect enough. But with my new way of thinking, I've done not one, but two photoshoots, one a lifestyle photoshoot and the other a fitness one! I had a blast at both! I was nervous and it definitely felt a bit weird, but in the end I really enjoyed myself.

Now, if I want to do something, even if it seems scary, I just do it. I take the steps I need to take to get started, then I let it unfold as it will. Sometimes the unfolding seems ugly and disappointing, and that's okay. I let myself feel disappointed and then forgive myself and ask myself what I learned from the experience. This exercise helps me appreciate how interesting the lesson was.

Are you open to growth in your life? Try doing something scary. Take a step into the unknown and let yourself be open to what comes. Maybe there's a course you've always wanted to take. Maybe you feel like you want to write a book. Maybe you want to change careers. Whatever it is start the journey without worrying about everything that needs to be done. Just do one task a day that will bring you closer to what you want to achieve. It's important to just take it one little bit at a time.

I took small steps when I opened my studio. Some days I focused on pricing exercise equipment. Other days I did Google searches to see what other studios were doing so I could get my creative juices flowing. And then on other days I would look for affordable (or free) courses to try to learn as much as I could about running a fitness business. If I had known exactly what needed to be done to open a studio before I began this adventure, I never would have started and would have missed out on some of the greatest experiences, lessons, and people in my life.

Overthinking almost always leads to limiting yourself. Why would you ever limit yourself? Life is an adventure, and you should try out everything you desire. What's the worst thing that could happen? So what if it doesn't work out like you thought it would. Take the lessons you learned from it and keep growing! To me, not growing feels like rotting. It feels stagnant and boring. Maybe it also feels safe, but what's the point of just feeling safe for your whole life? Live your adventure and enjoy every part of it.

What excites you? Have you ever wanted to try something but decided not to because it was so far out of your comfort zone? My challenge to you is to just try it. Commit and then work for it. Is it a trip to some exotic place all on your own? Book the trip now! Always wanted to try one of those Spartan races? Sign up now! Whatever it is, commit to it while you're feeling scared and unsure and I guarantee you will find a way to make it happen. And if it doesn't, who the hell cares?

You only get this one life, so why not experience all you can? Have fun with yourself! What are you waiting for? It makes absolutely no sense to not do something that interests you, even if it scares the crap out of you right now. You just may discover that you always learn something, and if you let yourself be open enough, you'll even find the lesson interesting.

Unexpected things happen, and that's okay. It's exciting when you're open to growth.

★

Here's what you're "supposed" to do:
Be open to things happening how they happen,
not necessarily how you planned. Step out of your
comfort zone so you can grow as a person.
Evolution is survival, so keep evolving and
get excited about what's next.

★

Here's what I did:
I let go of trying to make things work out exactly
as planned. I let go of striving for safety.

★

How that worked out for me:
Amazingly well! I feel like I wasn't really living
until I learned to be open to whatever came my
way. It boosted my self-esteem and made
me less fearful of trying other things that
I was interested in but were scary.

★

What are you going to do?

Epic Fails

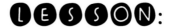:

**You have to fail if you want to learn and grow.
Failure can be viewed as bad, even devastating,
or it can be viewed as an adventure
that teaches you what not to do.**

Have you ever failed at something? Like in an epic way? If you haven't, you really need to try it! After the dust settles, you'll find that you didn't die and the world didn't come to an end. You'll dust yourself off and say, "Well, that sucked, but I got through it and am still here. Life goes on." You also learn some interesting lessons.

I remember the first time I felt like a failure. It was in kindergarten. I woke up feeling so excited. The day I had been waiting for had finally come! We were going to learn how to read! My parents could read, my big sister could read, and now I was going to read! My whole world was about to change.

I sat on the classroom carpet with my book, feeling proud that I was about to learn how to read. The book was called *Sis the Snake*. It was good! I liked Sis. He was a cool snake that was going to teach me how to read. When my first-ever reading lesson was over, I was dumbfounded. We were just given a lesson on how to read, yet I was not able to read all the books that I wanted to. What had happened? I was angry and frustrated with myself because I didn't leave that day being able to read everything. So from a very early age I was quite hard on myself. I didn't give up on reading, obviously, but I do have a tendency to give up on things that I'm not good at right away.

Failing is a great way to learn some powerful life lessons, but it can also become a problem if you feel like you're always failing. It can really put a damper on your mood. But here's the thing: it's most likely that you're not actually failing, you're just interpreting things the wrong way.

The closing down of my studio really taught me to not fear failure. When I had to close my doors, I thought that I had experienced the motherload of failure. All the time and money that I had invested had not paid off in the end. At first I thought that my world was going to come to an end and that there was no bigger failure than having to shut down a business that I had put so much into running. I felt embarrassed and disappointed in myself. But here's what's wonderful about life: it doesn't come to a complete stop when things don't work out like you wanted them to or expected.

I allowed myself a few days to feel sorry for myself and for the loss of something that I had put so much time, effort, and money into, then I examined what had happened and what I'd learned from the experience. Apparently, I am very good at training people and motivating them to take care of their health, but I suck at running a business.

Once I accepted this as my truth, opportunities to do what I love the most came my way. I was contacted by people who asked if I was interested in teaching and training at their gyms. I got offered jobs to do what I do best. I suddenly found myself in the exact situation I wanted to be in—I was living my dream! I was working full time as a fitness instructor and personal trainer, and I had (and still have) the absolute best clients in the world.

I had thought that having my own studio was my dream, but I learned that my real dream was to be able to work with people to improve their health without worrying about how I was going to make rent every month. I got out of my own way by letting go of my "failed" attempt at running my own studio, and when I did, what I had always wanted just came to me. The package looked a bit different from what I had pictured in my head, but my perfect situation presented itself without me feeling like I was fighting every step of the way and working 24/7. I finally felt like I got what I was chasing after.

When you're chasing something and feeling desperate to have it, it eludes you. Once you relax and let things unfold as they will, it's likely you'll get the outcome you were wanting, even if it looks a bit different from what you'd expected. Have you ever heard someone talk about how they met their soulmate when they weren't even looking for a relationship? Perhaps when we feel desperate for something we reek of that desperation, and it repels all chances of getting what we want. Cats are like that. When you try to get a cat to come to you, they tend to avoid you. The cat then usually goes to the one person who really doesn't want their attention and is doing their best to avoid eye contact!

Just because something doesn't turn out exactly as you pictured it in your head does not mean that you're a failure. Most things don't turn out as you pictured them. Even this book isn't what I had originally thought my book was going to be. Does that mean I failed? No! It means I've learned something. It means I started down one path and ended up on another path. It's an adventure!

I've learned not to label things as either successful or a failure. That's too black and white. The end result might not look exactly as you had pictured, but that doesn't mean that you failed—it means you found what you were looking for.

★

Here's what you're "supposed" to do:
Go ahead and fail. If you never fail,
you're not challenging yourself enough—you've set
the bar too low for how great you really are.

★

Here's what I did:
I avoided anything I thought I wouldn't be good
at so I could avoid failure. It was boring,
and I missed out on a lot. After years of always
being scared to challenge myself, I finally pushed
myself and experienced some epic fails.

★

How that worked out for me:
Great! I learned that if I failed I wouldn't die and the
world wouldn't explode. I learned powerful lessons
from my failures that allowed me to grow and
become more than I thought was possible.

★

What are you going to do?

It Really Doesn't Have to Be Perfect

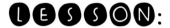:

Don't get caught up in trying to do everything perfectly. Letting go of having to be perfect lifts an enormous amount of pressure off you.

Perfection. Why do we strive for it? It's like setting ourselves up for failure because no matter how well we do something, it'll never be good enough for a perfectionist.

Somewhere along the line I decided that if it wasn't perfect, it was a failure that I should be punished for. There was no in-between for me. This belief created a lot of pressure and even more anger and frustration toward myself. For instance, if I had been "good" all day and hadn't eaten anything, but then had a slip and ate something, I'd decide that I had messed up and might as well keep going. This would lead to an all-out binge and possibly purging. Then I would beat myself up for having been so weak. Or if I missed a workout, I'd tell myself that I failed again and would always be a lazy, fat pig. Why was I so hard on myself?

So how did I get over it? A bit of it is still with me, but the voice in my head that loves to criticize me is way quieter. It used to be the dominant voice, but over the years I've learned to quiet her. With practice I learned to be more easygoing. Instead of beating myself up for having given in to the temptation of a cookie, I'd talk myself down by telling myself that it was a small slip, no big deal, and all I had to do was stop, dust myself off, and move on. This way of thinking wasn't easy in the beginning, though. Changing your thought patterns is never easy. As I was working on changing my thought patterns, I really liked the feeling of letting things go. So much pressure was lifted off me. But it was also a bit scary. Letting go of former thoughts felt like letting go of control, and that was frightening. Thankfully, I was so done with the hate in my head that I just pushed on and kept practicing being a bit nicer to myself. It became easier, but to this day I still have a need to keep myself somewhat in check. I'm not as strict with myself as I used to be, though, and one of the great payoffs of this new way of treating myself is that I actually started to feel happier.

Striving for perfection can make you feel so overwhelmed that you give up entirely or don't even start. Trying to do everything perfectly has held me back in the past because as soon as I found out that I couldn't do it perfectly, I gave up on it. I probably missed out on a lot of fun by limiting myself in that way. There were things that I chose to not even try because I was sure I'd be bad at it. Who cares if you're bad at something?

What if you had a super fun time at being bad at something? You don't have to be perfect at something in order to get joy out of it. Stop overthinking everything and just do what you can to keep moving forward.

Take this book, as an example. If I told myself that it had to be perfect, I would have never started it. Does that mean that I'm not having fun writing it? No! I've really enjoyed the process even when I felt like I was failing at it.

There is no "perfect" way to do anything. Perfection exists naturally. How things unfold and turn out is exactly how they were supposed to happen even if the outcome seems wrong. You can't be black or white about the world around you. Look for the lessons. Ask why something happened and what you learned from it rather than why it didn't go the way you expected it to. You have to practice changing your thinking. Try asking yourself if you'd demand the same level of perfection from someone you love. If the answer is no, then don't put that pressure on yourself.

Perfection is whatever is. Whatever you do, it's perfect. You might not think it is because it doesn't quite measure up to what you had in mind, but in actuality, it really is perfect. Instead of getting down on yourself because you didn't do something the way you thought you should, find the perfection in what you did.

★

Here's what you're "supposed" to do:
Don't expect everything to work out perfectly.
Don't shame yourself when things don't go
as planned. Don't limit yourself by not trying
things that you don't think you'll be good at.

★

Here's what I did:
I expected perfection and beat myself up
when things didn't go as planned. I shied away
from trying anything that I thought I might not be
good at. If I did try something new and I wasn't
good at it right away, I gave up. If it wasn't perfect,
I considered it a total disaster and continued
down the path of self-destruction until I
almost couldn't stand myself or my life.

★

How that worked out for me:
Not good. I missed out on opportunities to grow
and have fun. I felt irritated with myself
most of the time because, in my eyes,
what I did was never "perfect." I never felt happy
or at ease with myself. I felt like I was fighting
a losing battle. I felt like I was just waiting

to mess up again so I could prove to myself
what a worthless piece of crap I was.
Those were dark times.

★

What are you going to do?

BODY

♡

SETTING THE GROUNDWORK FOR SUCCESS

It's time to start the journey to a healthy and happy life! In this next section we'll dive into some fitness and nutrition guidance for getting healthy, but first we need to talk about how to set yourself up for success.

If you really want to make a change in your life, you must have a reason that's super important to you—something personal that has a big effect on your life. Trying to give something up because you know you "should" isn't going to be enough to motivate you to make a lasting change. In fact, it becomes a frustrating fight that you're probably always going to lose. Want change? You need a reason big enough to make that change worthwhile. You need to find your pain. If you can't come up with a strong enough reason, if you can't feel enough pain in not changing, you're probably not ready to make that change.

When I hit my rock bottom, I felt that pain and I made that change.

Here's what happened: I slowly started feeling better. I experienced little victories here and there, and that started the momentum. I kept moving forward, and the momentum kept increasing. I finally got to a point where proper nutrition and exercise were nonnegotiable parts of my life, and I took time to feel gratitude for what I had been through and for all the benefits of my new healthy lifestyle. It was literally life changing for me.

Improving your health can be uncomplicated, but if you overthink it, it can become an all-consuming, frustrating obsession. Once again, the key is simplicity: take baby steps. Start with simple changes first. Eat whole foods (try to eliminate as much overly processed foods as possible). Drink more water. Sleep more. Simple changes can have a major effect on your life, so don't try to get everything perfect. Focus on making the small changes that you feel confident about doing. If you have a bad day where you eat junk, forget to drink water, or don't get enough sleep, just dust yourself off and keep moving forward. We all have days that aren't ideal, but that just keeps life interesting. Can you imagine if every day was perfect? Can you imagine how boring that would get?

Treat your body in a healthful way and your body will naturally begin to improve. Your body wants nothing more than to survive and be healthy, but it doesn't have a chance if you don't care for it properly. Here's a tip to help keep things simple: Care for your body the same way you'd care for someone you love who is totally dependent on you and your decisions.

If you're a parent, you know what it means to care for someone you love more than life itself. Or maybe you have a pet that you love more than life. Perhaps you're caring for an aging parent who depends on your help. Think about how you feel about the person or animal you're caring for: you'd do anything they need to keep them healthy. You need to learn how to apply that same amount of care to yourself! And before you even think it, don't let yourself believe for one second that taking care of yourself is selfish. The only way you can be 100 percent there for those you love is to make sure you are the healthiest you can be.

Before we get into how to make these changes, there are two steps that you need to do to set yourself up for success: you need to set your goals and prepare for setbacks. Goals are important for giving you clear direction and keeping you on track. Preparing for setbacks is important because in real life, setbacks happen.

Let's get set up for success!

Time to Set Some Goals

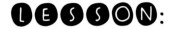 :

**Your goals need to be clear
and have a deep emotional meaning to you
if you really want to achieve something.**

We've all heard it before: you need to have clear goals if you want to achieve something. Not everyone knows how to set proper goals, however.

Stating that you want to start a fitness program to lose weight or get healthy is not a goal. It's a wish, and one that usually gets pushed aside because you think you're too busy with everything else in your life. Your goal needs to be specific, and it needs to evoke an emotional response from you. Typically, you're not feeling a lot of pleasure when you're working out. If you did, everyone would be doing it! So, the trick is to find the deep pain that will be relieved by sticking to a regular workout plan. You need to figure out what exactly your pain is—people will only dedicate time and effort to things that either provide pleasure or ease pain.

I had hit my rock bottom. That was the pain I needed to feel in order to make myself take action. What's your pain point? What needs to happen to make you decide that your current life isn't good enough for you anymore? What's your deep reason for wanting to become healthier? What will make you realize that you've had enough of dreaming about it and that now is the time for action? Is it so you can be around longer for your kids? Is it so you won't become a burden on your loved ones when your body breaks down? Is it because you're sick of feeling depressed and unhappy about your body? Is it because you feel like you've tried everything and nothing has worked and you're desperate to find something that does?

You need to dig deep and find the pain!

STEP 1: HAVE A GOAL!

Your goal must resonate deeply with you. You need to believe with all your heart that if you don't start working toward it that there will be immediate and intense pain. You need to believe that by taking action toward your goal you will feel immense pleasure. To really dig deep and find the pain, spend some time alone and let yourself feel the pain associated with being unhealthy and unhappy with how your body feels. You'll want to write down the real reasons you want to work on your health. Go deep!

Here's what you do:

- Sit somewhere where you won't be interrupted and think about how you're feeling about your physical and mental health.

- Write down what comes to mind and let yourself experience all the feelings that come with it. Get emotional. You need to get to the point where you truly feel like you've had enough of your current lifestyle and habits. Making changes won't happen long term if you aren't fired up about making them.

- Write down your goal.

- Write down at least three reasons why this goal is important to you.

- For each of those reasons, write down three reasons why those reasons are important to you.

See where I'm going?

Remember, you need to feel emotion when you think of your goal. As humans, we react to emotion, not common sense. Something can make total sense to you, such as losing weight to help your health, but you won't act on it unless you feel emotion when you think about it. Find your pain! Once you find your pain, you're ready to start. If you aren't feeling the pain, do not move onto the next step until you do.

STEP 2: KEEP REMINDING YOURSELF OF YOUR GOAL!

Now that you have established your goals, you need to keep them alive. You'll want to write them down DAILY.

Write your goals every day as if they've already happened and you're living the dream. For instance, write down how great it feels now that you've made healthy eating and exercise a priority and you suddenly have lots of energy. Write about how much your life has improved! Make it real! Make it emotional! If you fully engage in the exercise, it will inspire you like you won't believe. It will keep you motivated to keep moving toward your goal.

Do this daily first thing in the morning and/or before bed. Writing down your goals helps ingrain them in your mind, which leads to action without having to force yourself.

If you want to reach your goals, you have to become obsessed with them. Write them down, think about them every chance you get, and really get them entrenched in your mind. The human brain is amazing. Load it up with thoughts about what you want your life to be, and before long, you'll start taking the actions needed that will lead you to your goals. Believe to your core that you will achieve your goals even if you don't know exactly how.

It's amazing what focusing on something can do. Try this: Close your eyes and try to think of every red item in your room. Now open your eyes and count how many red objects there are. Probably a lot more than you pictured in your head, right? That's because when you focus on something, you see it. Here's another example: Have you ever decided to buy a certain make of car and then all of a sudden you see that exact car everywhere? It's not that these cars just suddenly showed up. They were there all along but now that you're focused on that particular make and model, you see it. Make sense?

We can only notice so much in our environment. If we noticed everything, we'd have sensory overload, so the brain filters out what's not important to us. Once you focus on something, however, your brain allows you to see it. Try it the next time you're searching for something in a cluttered drawer. At first you probably won't see it, so try saying the name of the item in your head. You'll find it! Focus and you'll see what you need to see.

It's true with goals as well. If you focus on your goals, you will begin seeing opportunities for achieving them. It's amazing! Write down your goals every single day. Get your brain focused on what you want so you can see all the ways toward getting it. But remember that training your mind to focus on the life you want can be difficult at first, especially if you've been in a negative state for some time. Change doesn't happen overnight, and it's going to take work.

Don't get discouraged. There will be setbacks, and you need to be ready for them. Don't be scared. Setbacks keep life interesting and keep you growing.

Indulging in Setbacks: Conversations with My Scale

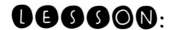**:**

Don't let some random number decide whether you're good or bad. A setback is only a setback if you get stuck in it.

Here are some conversations I've had (and sometimes still have) with my scale:

- *What the BLEEP? That can't be right!*

- *Ooh! Down a few pounds! I love you, and together we are awesome!*

- *Hold still while I kick the crap out of you.*

- *Come on, give me a good number today.*

- *You better show me a good number today!*

- *That's it! I'm throwing you out!*

- *Time to replace you with a scale that actually works.*

- *Stupid new scale! Why are you weighing two pounds higher than my old one?*

- *That can't be right. Must be water retention.*

- *That can't be right. Must be getting my period.*

- *That can't be right.*

It can be easy to give your power to something outside of yourself (like the bathroom scale!), as doing so allows you to blame something rather than looking inside yourself and trying to fix what's not working. For me, my anger was directed at the scale, but my real anger was at myself for not doing what needed to be done to get the outcome I wanted.

The word *setback* implies that you're moving backward and essentially failing. I've had many setbacks in my life, and I used to get so mad at myself for having "failed" again. It was my all-or-nothing attitude kicking in, and I nearly always ended up in tears.

Recently, though, I've learned that setbacks can be quite valuable. Consider setbacks as revisiting something you used to like in order to see if you like it now. You revisit the behavior, you get feedback, then you decide whether you want to continue down that path. I've found that giving up my unhealthy habits is sort of like breaking up with someone, then getting back together with them for a night. In my case, I used to beat myself up for revisiting old habits, and I'd quite often be stuck for a bit. But once I gave myself permission to forgive myself, I found I was able to move on more quickly.

Have you ever abstained from drinking, then found yourself out with friends one night getting drunk? How do you feel the next day? In your worst case scenario, you have another drink to cure your hangover. Your best case scenario is that you feel horrible, and that horrible feeling reminds you why you don't drink anymore. If nothing else, setbacks remind you of where you don't want to be. It doesn't mean you'll never revisit prior behavior, it just means that you won't make it a regular part of your day.

Losing the fight can feel frustrating, but fighting to not lose the fight can be exhausting, so for my life I decided that setbacks would happen and the best way for me to deal with them was to only let them happen for a short period of time. I put a limit on how long they could last. I'd allow myself to feel frustrated, angry, and sad (or whatever other emotions came up) for a day, week, or however long I needed. What worked for me was to give myself permission to stumble and know that it was part of what I needed to fully heal. Giving myself this permission relieved some of the pressure, as I was letting myself be human.

So, let's drop the word setback from our vocabulary. Replace "setback" with "revisit." Be kind to yourself. Tell yourself that you had a revisit because you just wanted to make sure it wasn't a habit you might like to let back into your life. Also, give yourself permission to perhaps revisit it again in the future if you decide you want to. When you give yourself permission to do something, it takes the power away from the situation and puts it in your hands. For me, if I decide I'm not allowed to do something, that something suddenly becomes very seductive. If I decide I'm allowed to do something, that something suddenly doesn't seem as fun. I think it's a quirk that we all have. We desperately want the thing we've been told we're not allowed to have. It's not as fun if we're given permission to do it.

What keeps me coming back to living a healthy lifestyle? My mindset change and how I feel about life. When I don't take proper care of myself, I start feeling bad; I start feeling anxious and depressed again. It gives me a glimpse of how miserable I was before and reminds me that I truly do want to be happy and excited about life. I literally tell myself, "I CANNOT go back there. I CANNOT go back to that dark pit of despair." And what would be the point if I did? What would it accomplish for me? Nothing. It turns me into a self-isolated, angry, sad mess.

I made the decision to let myself experience "revisits" without judgment. I still get down on myself occasionally, but I look for the lesson. Most times the lesson is that perfect kick in the ass to get me back on track.

Here are some tricks to help keep you on the healthy path:

- Get rid of the scale and measuring tapes if you find yourself obsessing over the numbers.

- Avoid tight-fitting clothing. If you bought clothes at a particularly low weight, get rid of them.

- Avoid mirrors on those hard days when you're feeling down about yourself.

- When looking in a full-length mirror, tilt it so that you can't see your face. You'll be amazed by how you look at your body when you can't see your face attached to it.

- Stay away from websites that promote unhealthy lifestyles. Take a break from social media completely, if possible.

- Find balance in your highs and lows.

Now, if you've previously been practicing unhealthy habits to lose weight, this simple plan may not seem like it's working at first. If you've been consuming unhealthy foods, not exercising, not drinking enough water or getting enough sleep, it's most likely that your hormones are out of balance. Don't worry! If you stay consistent with healthy living your body will do it's best to correct these issues. It will take time, though. Make healthy changes and stick with them for a minimum of three months. I know that three months sounds like a long commitment, so just take it one day at a time. Most people begin to see and feel a difference after this time period. Some will notice changes sooner, and some may have to stick with it just a bit longer before they notice the positive results, but it will happen!

★

Here's what you're "supposed" to do:
Get rid of your scale and stop putting so much
stock in random numbers that don't tell you
anything about your health. After a setback,
get back up, dust yourself off, and move on.

★

Here's what I did:
I pursued a long-term relationship with my scale.
I took setbacks as a measure of my self-worth
and let them feed the fire of self-hatred I had.

★

How that worked out for me:
How good or bad of a day I was going to have
became dependent on what the scale told me,
so I had a lot of really bad days. I mentally abused
myself by telling myself how lazy, ugly, and worthless
I was. I was a mess! I sometimes got stuck in the
setback and wasted too much valuable time
steeping in the negativity when I should have
been learning from the experience.

★

What are you going to do?

MAKING THE NUTRITION CONNECTION

Proper nutrition saved me. It changed everything. I fought eating proper nutrition for a long time, and the harder I fought, the worse things got. When I started to eat properly, my mind got healthy, and the rest fell into place. The hardest part for me was being brave enough to make friends with what I thought was the enemy: food.

In the end, it was simple: Small steps. Patience. Trust. Success!

Eating proper nutrition helps your mind work optimally. You're able to make sense of things. You're able to see happiness and hope. You're able to function and be productive. When I stopped obsessing so much over food and how I looked, it freed up so much of my time. I discovered my strengths and what made me happy and fulfilled, and it all started with food. This sounds so simple, but when you're in an unhealthy mental state, it is anything but. Proper nutrition can be uncomplicated. It only gets complicated when you listen to the messages that the diet industry is pumping out. Once again, the key is simplicity.

Our bodies are constantly changing—they break down and rebuild. But they can only rebuild out of what's put in. Put crap in your body and your body uses that crap to rebuild itself. It's like building a house: use crappy materials and end up with a house that has a leaky roof; use high-quality materials and you get a strong house that will stand the test of time. There may be issues here and there, but they're way less devastating.

So, what does a body need? It needs healthy carbs, proteins, and fats, enough water, enough sleep, and daily breaks from the chronic stress that most of us experience without even being that aware of it. This isn't to say that you have to be perfect all the time, as that's way too much pressure. You just need to work on the things that aren't optimal and be patient. As your body and brain start to get healthier, it gets easier.

It All Starts with Food

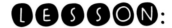:

Food is our most important medicine. Without proper nutrition, the body and mind break down and all that follows is misery and discomfort.

When I was at rock bottom, I hated my life so much. I dreaded every day. I'd wake up and, within seconds, be filled with anxiety. I wanted to escape from myself, but there's no breaking up with yourself—you're the one person you are stuck with for your entire life. So, I decided that I had to change how I was living.

I found a great nutrition course called Certified Sports Nutrition Advisor by Cory Holly (for more information, please visit the Resources section). I had heard Cory speak and decided to purchase his home study course and learn a bit about nutrition. As I studied it, something really spoke to me. It explained nutrition in a way that made sense to me, but did I believe it enough to apply it to myself? I was so tired of feeling depressed and ashamed about my body. Something had to give because I was not living a happy life, and I was only in my twenties; I had lots of life left to get through! When I got to my rock bottom, the decision became easier. I decided to follow the information in the course with the attitude of "what do I have to lose?" I would try it and if it didn't work out, I could go back to what I knew.

There were ups and downs and a few setbacks, but I kept up the fight because for the first time ever I saw a glimmer of the possibility of being at peace with myself and actually living a happy life that I could be excited about.

Here's how I started: I planned my meals. I chose healthy foods and put them on my menu. I cut out sugar, and I slowly cut out everything with chemicals. No more sugar-free/fat-free frankenfoods for me. Sure, the calories in those types of foods were low, but the chemical shitstorm they created in my body was destroying my body and mind. Changing the way I ate allowed my body to get leaner. Plus, my asthma and allergies went away, my mental state improved, and my energy skyrocketed!

I was quite skeptical in the beginning, but I was astonished when changing my nutrition actually worked! It didn't happen overnight, but slowly I started feeling better. I didn't feel as depressed, and my anxiety wasn't as extreme. I was acutely aware of these changes. I think being so desperate to be happy made me more sensitive to the tiny changes that started happening. I could see the light at the end of the tunnel.

And with my increased energy, I began enjoying my workouts. I felt great joy in how strong I was becoming. Suddenly weight loss became a nice side effect of something I really loved doing, which helped me to trust food and understand that optimal health comes from feeding my body what it needs. I discovered the power of eating proper food! It was so simple!

Soon, my love/hate relationship with food turned into a respectful one. Food wasn't the enemy, misinformation was. Learning and practicing proper nutrition and exercise changed my life. It took a long time for me to get to where I am now, but I did it and it was worth it.

Here are the steps I took to help improve my physical and mental health through proper nutrition:

I stopped looking at food as a calorie-filled enemy. You need to see food as a necessity for building a healthy body and mind. Keep reminding yourself that proper nutrition will bring you happiness. Trust me!

I stopped making certain foods off-limits. When something is off-limits, you'll just want it more. Even unhealthy choices can fit into a healthy plan that doesn't lead to weight gain. I have a cheat day once a week where I let myself indulge in whatever I feel like. But be careful that you don't binge. And if you do, stop, dust yourself off, and start again. This step takes some practice and may take time to master, so be patient!

I found reputable sources of information about nutrition. For example, I listen to Shawn Stevenson's podcast, *The Model Health Show* (visit the Resources section for more information). He went through an unbelievable health transformation and understands the connection between nutrition and optimal health. He's very inspiring and does his research.

Achieving a healthy body is something we can all do. It's not always easy, but it is simple. In fact, it's so simple that most people don't believe that it can possibly work. I was one of those people. Focus on eating healthy whole foods, avoiding processed crap, exercising moderately and consistently, drinking enough water, and getting good quality sleep. Simple, but again, not always easy. You have to be prepared to work a bit and get a little uncomfortable. Making changes may be uncomfortable, but stick with it because the results are well worth the effort.

When I look back at who I once was, one word comes to mind: pathetic. I don't mean this in a mean way, I just mean that I was so sad and so tired and the life I lived was just so damned depressing. Since getting my nutrition under control I've become happy and content with my life. I find joy in small things. I don't feel the need to impress people as much. I'd rather be happy than always trying to be something I'm not. I don't feel like I need to prove anything to anybody. I'm more concerned with being my true authentic self (I didn't even know who that was until I started eating properly!). Food! It's so simple! The answer was there all along, and I fought it so hard so I could win at being miserable.

If you're struggling with nutrition, I challenge you to commit to even just one week of eating healthfully. If that seems overwhelming, commit to just one day! You may even wish to hire a nutritionist or dietitian, but make sure they don't represent any particular brand because they might have their own agenda. Pay close attention to how you feel and how you think. I recommend keeping a journal because sometimes the positive changes are quite subtle, and you may not remember them. After that first week (or day) is over, push yourself to keep going another week (or day). As time passes, you're going to be surprised by how much better you feel.

★

Here's what you're "supposed" to do:
Eat a balanced diet of healthy whole foods and have respect for what the food does for your body.

★

Here's what I did:
At first, I avoided food as much as possible and used things like diet pop and cigarettes to curb my appetite. It took me a while, but I eventually made friends with food and learned to have a deep appreciation and respect for it.

★

How that worked out for me:
Not so good. Depression and anxiety were my normal mental state, and I berated myself daily. I was hardly living. Once I learned about proper nutrition, though, it completely changed my life. I felt like a fog had lifted and I was able to truly enjoy life.

★

What are you going to do?

Extreme Dieting

TRIGGER WARNING:
EXTREME DIETING; MENTAL HEALTH

LESSON:

**Most diets on the market are meant to put
money in their pockets rather than help you
with your health and body composition.
The diet industry wants your money,
and it doesn't care that it's destroying lives.**

Are you looking for that magic pill or magic program that's going to give you the body you want?

Stop looking! It doesn't exist. There is no magic when it comes to taking proper care of your body and achieving a healthy body composition. Advertisers for these types of products are very clever, though. They know what language to use to entice people into trying their products. Even with all my experience and education I still sometimes get tempted to try the latest "research-backed" pill/program/diet.

A few diets I've tried include:

- Calorie counting
- Elimination diet: eliminate as much food as possible
- Low-calorie microwave dinners. They were so

gross and looked so sad. I was so sad. I got really tired of being sad.

- Plans where you have "two shakes a day and a sensible dinner." What does a sensible dinner even look like after a day where you only drank two disgusting shakes?

- The potato and ketchup diet. Nothing but potatoes smothered in ketchup. It turns out if you're putting ketchup on your food, it's pretty much the same as pouring pure sugar on it.

- The all-rice diet. Part of this was because I was super broke, so I bought a huge bag of rice and lived off it. I'd make savory rice for main meals and then sweet rice for dessert. Sweet rice was rice sprinkled with calorie-free sweetener and cinnamon.

- The popcorn and cheese slice diet. I'd microwave a bag of popcorn and then tear up a no-name cheese product slice (I couldn't afford Kraft Singles), eat it, then go to the gym to work it off.

- And lastly, the cigarette and diet pop diet. I smoked when I was hungry and drank diet pop to make me feel full. Genius!

First, the bad news: there is no miracle product or diet plan that will magically get the job done.

But here's the good news: you can stop letting the diet industry confuse you. For some, this sounds like bad news because you get to a point where you're desperate for a miracle product or diet plan. I know this firsthand. It's actually good news, however, because you can give yourself permission to stop wasting your time and money on stuff that's not going to work.

Many people seem to think that getting healthy is complicated and out of reach, which is what the diet industry wants us to think so we buy their "miracle" products. I used to think that there was some secret or magical way to lose the weight, and I was always looking for the next great thing to make me into the person I wanted to be. I assumed that it would be a complicated process because there was so much conflicting information being broadcasted.

Don't feel bad if you are confused as to what's healthy and what's not. It's made to feel complicated and out of reach for a reason. The diet industry is a multibillion-dollar industry, and it depends on people being confused, frustrated, and ready to try anything (and spend anything) to achieve their health and fitness goals. Every time you see a new diet that's supposed to be the answer, there's a company behind it that's trying to get as much money as they can. People don't know what to do! Low carb? Low fat? All protein? This shake? This program? That pill? There's so much conflicting information that people just want to be told what to do because they've been made to feel that it's too complicated to understand properly. The diet industry confuses us into thinking that it's impossible to get the results we want on our own.

The problem with most diets is that they are too extreme and cut out too many nutrients. When you do extreme diets, your weight is not the only thing that is affected. Both your body and brain need nutrients to function properly. Not getting proper nutrients for your brain can lead to depression and anxiety. Your hormones are also affected, which can lead to depression and a damaged metabolism. And if you're feeling depressed and anxious all the time, you'll probably start searching out comfort foods for a little bit of pleasure. You want success on a diet? Then you need to choose a plan that you can stick with for the long run. It's all about consistency.

The hardest part of dieting is figuring out how many calories you should be eating. Luckily, there are skilled professionals that can help. Make sure you talk to someone with proper education who is not trying to sell you any kind of product.

Your body is your own personal research product. Every single body is different. What works for one person may not work for another person, so you need to experiment on yourself. You need to find what foods work well for you as well as what kind of physical activity works well for you. I've tried vegetarianism. I've tried high-protein diets. I've tried keto diets. What I found worked for me was a balance of carbs, proteins, and fats. I seem to operate best when I don't go extreme with anything. I know people who operate best on a keto diet, or as a vegan, or with intermittent fasting. We are all different.

The way you discover what's best for you is to keep track of how you are feeling physically and mentally. Learn to listen to your body and read the cues it's giving you. Keep a journal and note your energy levels, your mood, your menstrual cycle, your sex drive, and your overall attitude about life. For women, if your menstrual cycle is off, that's an indicator that something in your diet may be wrong. (Note: If you are experiencing cycle irregularities, please visit your doctor and get a full blood panel done. Quite often hormonal issues are caused by poor diet, but hormonal issues can also be an indicator of illness, so you should talk to your doctor.)

Try different whole foods to see what makes you feel the most energetic and the happiest. This can take a bit of time, but it's worth it. Be patient and kind to yourself and I promise that you'll reach the goal of being happy, healthy, and truly enjoying life!

★

Here's what you're "supposed" to do:
Find a way of eating and exercising that makes you feel on top of your world. Eat natural, whole foods. Avoid the "lose fat fast" gimmicks promoted by the diet industry.

★

Here's what I did:
At first, I fell for the gimmicks and tried all the stuff that promised to make me skinny. When I finally stopped, I experimented with different ways of eating and found what made me feel like a properly functioning, happy, energetic human being.

★

How that worked out for me:
I was depressed from being malnourished, and any weight I lost came back and brought more with it. Diets typically aren't sustainable long term. Once I gave up those diets, my life changed. It made me excited about life, which made me a more productive person who no longer longed to be "normal" like everyone else.

★

What are you going to do?

Foods That Talk

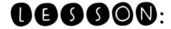:

**Eating junk food will never satisfy your cravings.
Eating junk will actually increase your cravings.**

The cheesecake called my name. At first, it was a whisper, but then it got louder. It got so loud that I couldn't drown it out and there was only one thing I could do: kill that piece of cheesecake by eating it.

Has this ever happened to you? Do certain foods talk to you? For me, it's usually something sweet, or Chicago-style popcorn, or dates, or ice cream. Sometimes it's cheese and cheese's best friend, wine. Why do certain foods talk to us?

The answer has to do with calories.

It's no secret that if you cut calories, you do lose weight. What happens when you restrict calories for too long, however, is that your body adapts to less energy coming in by learning how to store fat more efficiently. You then have to keep lowering your calories as your body adapts. Can you see the problem with this?

This is not a sustainable plan. What you eat affects your hormones and your hormones do a plethora of things in your body including telling your body when to store fat, how much fat to store, and when to release fat to be used as energy. An example I like to use with my calorie-conscious clients is this: Take two people and put them both on a daily 2,000-calorie diet. One person eats nothing but highly processed food. The other eats a diet of real whole foods. Even though they are on the same number of calories, you'll see two dramatically different bodies and minds. Food affects absolutely everything about you (for more about calories, visit the Resources section). The quality of food is what matters, and we were never meant to consume highly processed, chemically filled foods. If you can't find a certain food or its ingredients in nature, don't eat it.

Something I've learned since I started bodybuilding is that there is an inverse relationship between lowered calories and "talking" food. As calories go down, food's voice gets louder and more persistent. Food always spoke loudly to me when I was younger and was trying to starve myself into being skinny. At the time I just figured that I was weak and had no self-control. I thought that all I had to do was practice more self-control to reach my goal, but I'd fail every time and end up bingeing on something and hating myself even more.

I now know why those foods screamed at me and that giving in had nothing to do with self-control or being a "good" person. The body is very smart, and its driving force is survival. When you go on a low-calorie diet and start rapidly losing weight, your body sees this as a threat to its existence and starts sending out signals to find food. Specifically, it drives you to find high-calorie foods so that it can store as much energy as possible to get through the famine. This means that your metabolism slows down and no matter how low you drop your calories, your body will store them as fat so you can survive. This mechanism has been built into us since the beginning of time, something that is beneficial in times of famine, but not so much when we can eat food at any time.

Do you ever wonder why it's so easy to eat a large amount of junk food without feeling full? If you're like me, you've probably eaten way more than you meant to when deciding to treat yourself to a bag of chips, or popcorn, or whatever snack you're craving. This type of junk food has tons of calories but very few valuable nutrients. In an attempt to top up nutrients, your body will drive you to keep eating until you get the proper nutrients, but this will never happen with junk food. It's called junk for a reason. You might be able to power through an entire Costco bag of Chicago-style popcorn, but when was the last time you had the urge to eat an entire Costco bag full of apples?

When food is talking loudly to you, you are most likely deficient in something. If you're on a low-calorie diet, you're going to be deficient in some nutrients, which is why you have the cravings. It's your instinct driving you to eat to survive. You can try to ignore it, but it's difficult to ignore your need for survival. People feel like they're bad or out of control because they have these strong cravings. But the cravings are your survival mechanism, and you can't turn that off, which is why balance in diet is essential for physical and mental health.

It takes a lot of strength and courage to ignore the warped messages your mind is sending you about empty calories and to trust that eating the proper food will make everything better. When I changed my eating habits, I set a time limit. I promised myself I'd commit to a whole month of improving my nutrition, as that seemed doable for me. If a month sounds too long for you, perhaps you can commit to a week, or maybe just one day. To make changes you need to get the momentum rolling, and success in something will do just that.

Commit to an achievable goal and watch for the results. I told myself that if after a month of nutritious eating things weren't working out, I could go back to my old habits and keep starving myself and living a miserable existence. After that month, though, I knew there was no turning back. I was interested in and excited about life. I was in a great mood most of the time. I wasn't completely derailed whenever something stressful happened. There was no way in hell I was ever going to go back to the miserable world I had created in my head when I wasn't eating properly.

Think of it this way: if you own a super-expensive luxury car, you're going to want to put the best gas and other car fluids in it, and you're going to take that precious car in for its regular maintenance appointments. Treat your body like you'd treat that super-expensive luxury car. Put the best things in it, take it out on a regular basis so it doesn't seize up, and keep up on regular maintenance. In other words, eat food that's real. Drink about one ounce of water per pound of body weight. Get seven to nine hours of quality sleep per night. Fit some physical activity in on most days of the week. That's it. The result will be a fine-tuned machine that will last a lifetime.

★

Here's what you're "supposed" to do:
Don't go on extreme, unsustainable diets.
Instead, feed yourself properly so food
doesn't start "talking" to you.

★

Here's what I did:
I starved myself until I couldn't drown out the voices
of the food. I put myself on every possible diet I
could find with the belief that one had to work.

★

How that worked out for me:
Not good. Years and years of the starving/bingeing/
purging/hating-myself-with-a-blind-passion cycle.
I lost weight, then gained it all back plus more,
which spiraled me into a deep depression.

★

What are you going to do?

My (Partial) Breakup with Alcohol

LESSON:

**If you're constantly looking for an escape
and are using substances like alcohol to achieve it,
there's something out of balance in your life.
More substance abuse leads to more imbalance.
The hole just keeps getting deeper.**

At a very young age I got to have a tiny bit of alcohol on special occasions such as Christmas and Thanksgiving. It was the Swedish influence on my dad's side. There's a picture of me at around three or four years old in my onesie with a tiny glass of rum and coke. So cute . . . or maybe a red flag.

I was about ten when my friend and I discovered some unopened beer left on a trail by our school and decided to try it. My friend opened the bottle using the fence (she was so crafty!), and we had a bit. I felt guilty about it for years after. Like super guilty—I prayed and promised God that I would never drink or smoke ever.

But that didn't last! At age fourteen, my friends and I usually figured out ways to get alcohol to drink on the weekends. I loved drinking. I loved the escape. I loved that feeling of being a bit out of control and irresponsible. This would be the case for many, many years.

For me, alcohol was my escape, my way to relax and get out of my head. It was my friend. I had no idea how trapped it was keeping me. Alcohol is a depressant. You may feel good in the moment, but the next day you feel down and tired and just want to feel good again, which typically leads to more drinking. It can be a vicious cycle when it gets out of control.

I knew I was drinking more than I should, a habit that went on for years. I kept thinking about cutting back. I thought about just drinking on the weekends or even just every other day. Unfortunately, by the time I got to the end of my day, all I could think about was having a glass of wine. I just wasn't ready. I told myself, "If this is wrong, I don't want to be right!" When you're not ready to make a change, it becomes a lot harder to make it. You feel like it's a battle that cannot be won. I didn't consider myself a raging alcoholic. I didn't miss work because of my drinking, and I was responsible and reliable. I didn't destroy my relationships because of my drinking, although I probably came close. Thus, there was really no great reason for me to give it up.

Then came bodybuilding. I decided I wanted to compete; I decided to get WAY out of my comfort zone. I hired a coach, and she asked me to submit a food diary. After she read it, she asked me if I always drank that much. She wasn't judging, she just wanted to know. I told her that I drank two to three big glasses of wine every night and usually more on the weekends. The plan she had for me included alcohol, but only on my cheat day. I really didn't know if I'd be able to do that, but I had invested the money for a coach and had a huge goal—to walk out on a stage with other beautiful women, wearing next to nothing and having a group of people judge me on how I looked, and boy did that keep me motivated to stick to the plan. It was easier than I thought it would be to cut down my drinking to once a week, as I loved waking up on weekdays with a clear head and energy to burn!

After a few competitions I decided that I wanted to do a dry-prep—I'd drink no alcohol for three to four months. I never thought I could do it, but I was genuinely curious to see how cutting alcohol would affect my physique, so I was highly motivated and was super happy with the results. The training became easier because I had more energy, and I was able to build more muscle by eliminating alcohol (for more information, visit the Resources section).

I still drink alcohol now and then, but I don't love it as much as I used to. I've learned that the short time spent feeling "good" after a few drinks is not worth feeling horrible the rest of the time. Also, who wants to be the annoying drunk who people try to avoid? Gone are the days when I was counting the hours until I could sit down with my glass of wine. I was ready to give it up.

★

Here's what you're "supposed" to do:
If you're going to drink, drink responsibly.

★

Here's what I did:
I drank irresponsibly. When I wasn't drinking, I was thinking about drinking. I was always looking forward to the escape at the end of the day.

★

How that worked out for me:
Not good. I was depressed and anxious and self-conscious about the possibility of my clients smelling the previous night's alcohol on me during 6 a.m. sessions and classes. There were times when I was teaching spin and was just hoping and praying that I wouldn't throw up.
Sadly, this felt normal to me.

★

What are you going to do?

UNDERSTANDING WHAT YOU EAT: WHAT THE HELL ARE MACROS?

Somewhere along the way people lost their instinctual connection to food. Calories suddenly seemed like the most important aspect for trying to improve body composition. Weight gain/loss became all about calories in versus calories out. The problem with this way of thinking, however, is that it doesn't take into account the importance of balanced macronutrients.

I first learned about macronutrients, or macros, when I took Cory Holly's nutrition course. Even after learning about them, though, I tended to focus on calories since it seemed like all the "experts" agreed that losing weight came down to counting them. It wasn't until I started training for bodybuilding competitions that I really started to understand that the types of foods you eat are even more important than the total number of calories consumed. All food has calories, but not all foods have the same effect on your body composition.

So, what are macronutrients? Macronutrients are basically carbs, proteins, and fats.

Let's take a look at each in turn!

The "F" Word: Fat Is Not the Enemy

ⓁⒺⓈⓈⓄⓃ:

We need fat to survive and thrive!
Proper fat intake will improve body composition.

Do you remember in the '80s when an infomercial lady adopted the catch phrase "fat makes you fat"? Remember that? Remember all the low-fat and fat-free products that came on the market? I sure do! I embraced the fat-free lifestyle a little too much. I was terrified of fat. Fat was the enemy.

Do you know what happened? The obesity epidemic started to explode. But how could this be? We cut fat out of our diets. Why aren't we all ultra-skinny super-models? Something didn't add up (for more on the obesity epidemic, see the Resources section).

As it turns out, our body needs fat to survive and thrive. If we don't get enough fat, our hormones become unbalanced, which leads to a myriad of problems!

Why do we need fat? Well, here are some facts you may not be aware of:

Your brain is mostly fat! It has the consistency of soft butter, which is why it's the only organ that is encased in its own hard shell. If you've ever gone on a low-fat diet, you've probably experienced some brain fog. That's because your brain needs healthy fats to operate at optimum levels.

You need fat so you can absorb the fat-soluble vitamins A, D, E, and K. These vitamins are important to good health, but if you cut out all the fat from your diet, you won't be able to absorb these vitamins properly. Without these important vitamins, you'll experience dry skin, weak and brittle nails, and dull hair that may start to fall out.

Fat helps regulate body temperature. If you've ever been on a low-fat diet, chances are you experienced being cold all the damn time.

Fat helps your immune system. With all we've experienced in the not-so-distant past, no one can argue that we need a strong immune system. I remember being sick pretty much all the time (like at least one cold every month) when I was starving my body of fat.

Fat also helps you feel full so you don't overeat. Have you ever noticed that you could easily eat an entire box of fat-free cookies and then still want to eat more? To make the cookies taste good and have an appealing texture, there is added sugar (sometimes artificial no-calorie sweeteners) but no fat.

Wait! Before you start eating all the fat in sight, you need to know that not all fats are created equal (see the

Resources section for more information). There are healthy fats and not-so-healthy fats, and then there are the truly damaging fats.

Healthy fats:

- Polyunsaturated fats such as fatty fish, flax seed, and plant-based liquid cooking oils such as olive, hemp, and avocado oil.

- Monounsaturated fats such as nuts, seeds, and avocados.

- Saturated fats (yup! These too have a place in a healthy diet . . . in moderation, of course) such as full-fat butter, cream, and cheese (hard cheese is higher in saturated fats than soft cheeses).

Some foods that are sources of healthy fat:

- Plant-based oils such as extra virgin olive, hemp, flax, and avocado
- Nut butters
- Real butter from grass-fed cows
- Full-fat yogurt
- Nuts and seeds
- Avocados
- Whole eggs
- Cheese (if you're watching your saturated fat intake, the softer cheeses have less saturated fat)

- Dark chocolate! Get the stuff that's at least 70 percent cocoa.

- Fatty fish such as salmon, trout, mackerel, sardines, and herring.

- Coconut and coconut oil. Coconuts and coconut oil are high in medium chain triglycerides (mct). They are metabolized differently, and some studies have shown that they can benefit people with Alzheimer's and even help burn belly fat (see the Resources section for more information).

As for unhealthy fats, there's just one super-bad one that you need to avoid completely: artificial trans fat. And—surprise, surprise—the unhealthy fat is the one that is made in a lab and not naturally occurring! These fats are created by pumping hydrogen molecules into vegetable oils. These are found in processed foods such as cookies, cakes, pizzas, and crackers, so check the labels. Here's the tricky thing, though. The FDA allows foods with 0.5 grams or less of trans fats per serving to be listed as trans-fat–free. But you're smarter than they are because you're going to read the ingredient label and look for the words "hydrogenated" or "partially hydrogenated." If you see those words, steer clear!

Fat is not the enemy! You can actually end up gaining more fat by avoiding healthy fats. Eat the proper ones and you'll have energy, a clear and focused mind, beautiful glowing skin, strong nails, and shiny hair. The right fats will keep you looking and feeling your best. I know this can feel scary and completely wrong, so start slowly by introducing a few healthy fats into your diet such as olive oil, nuts, or avocados and let yourself experience the magic of fats for yourself.

★

Here's what you're "supposed" to do:
Eat an appropriate amount of healthy fats.

★

Here's what I did:
I avoided fat like the plague.

★

How that worked out for me:
I was depressed, had dry hair and skin,
felt tired all the time, and got chubbier.

★

What are you going to do?

Where's the Beef? Facts About Protein
ⓁⒺⓈⓈⓄⓃ:
You need protein, but don't overdo it.

We need protein, but how much? Some people go to extremes with protein. Men and women who want to put on a lot of muscle start packing in protein. Protein builds muscle, right? It does, but just because you need a certain amount to build muscle does not mean that increasing it to as much as you can stomach will get you better results. Consuming too much protein can can be damaging to your kidneys if they are unhealthy.

So, how much do we need? A good rule, and it's easy to remember and figure out the numbers, is about 1 gram of protein per pound of body weight per day.

Here are some interesting facts about protein (also visit the Resources section for more information):

1 gram of protein has 4 calories, which is exactly the same as 1 gram of carbs. This is why calorie counting is not the best measure of a healthy diet. A diet of all carbs and no protein will lead to a very unhealthy body.

It helps reduce appetite. It takes a bit more time and effort for the body to break down protein, so you'll feel fuller for longer. If you've ever over eaten protein, you may have experienced some bloating and an increase in body temperature to a point where you break out in a sweat.

It increases muscle mass and strength. Protein is made up of amino acids and those amino acids are what our muscle cells use to repair and build more muscle cells. This does not mean that eating more than your body can use will make you more muscular. It'll just make you feel too full and may cause some excessive sweating.

It's good for your bones. There have been studies that have shown that people who eat more protein tend to maintain bone mass as they age. This is especially important for women because we tend to have a higher risk for osteoporosis after menopause.

It reduces cravings—even alcohol cravings! When I have a client who complains about cravings, more often than not when I look at their food diary their protein is too low. In fact, quite often before changing anything on anyone's diet, I have them add a bit of extra protein to it. I can't even count how many times I've had clients tell me that when they increased their protein their cravings just went away and their body composition started improving.

It boosts metabolism and increases fat burning! But again, before you go eat a steak the size of your head, remember that just because some is good does not mean that more is better. Protein has something that's known as the thermic effect. Basically, this means that more heat (a.k.a. more calorie burn) happens when you eat protein, which is why you may sweat after eating it.

It can lower blood pressure. There have been studies done that have shown that higher protein intake results in lower blood pressure. Remember, though, just because the right amount is effective does not mean that more is going to be more effective.

It helps your body repair itself after injury. If you work out, or even if you don't, at some point you will injure yourself. It's just a part of life if you venture out of bed every day. Protein provides the building blocks that your tissues need to repair themselves.

It does not harm healthy kidneys as long as you're not overconsuming it. If you have pre-existing kidney issues, you do have to be careful with your protein intake. (You must talk to your doctor about protein intake if you have kidney issues.) 0.8 to 1 gram of protein per pound of body weight is what you need to reap the benefits of it.

I find that most of my clients don't eat enough protein. There are a couple of main reasons for this. One, protein tends to be more expensive than other foods. Growing up, I often had mac and cheese with ketchup for dinner. Or Miracle Whip sandwiches. It was an affordable way to fill a hungry belly, but where was the protein? Another reason why people's protein intake can be a bit low is because it's much more convenient to eat carbs and fats. Just look at the snack aisle in the grocery store. Pretty much everything in it is carbs and fat. You might find some beef jerky, but chances are there's sugar added to it for better flavor, so it's definitely not an optimal source of protein.

Getting enough protein can be tricky, something I learned when I started bodybuilding. I found that my protein was often lower than where I wanted it to be, but I couldn't figure out how to increase protein without blowing my fat allowance. I found that egg whites are a great way to increase protein without adding fat. I add egg whites to my oatmeal for a protein-packed breakfast. I normally tell people to eat foods in their natural state (i.e., the whole egg because all the great vitamins and the fat needed to absorb them are in the yolk), but in a pinch, egg whites are a good way to get in more protein if needed. I also use protein shakes sparingly. I say sparingly because getting your nutrients from non-processed sources is best. At most, I'll have two protein shakes in a day. The key is to use it as a supplement, not as a replacement for real whole foods.

Some sources of protein are:

- Meat. Try to find meat that has been trimmed of excess fat. If you're eating poultry and you're really watching your fat intake, go for skinless. Confession: I once ordered myself a bucket of Kentucky Fried Chicken, ate a couple of pieces, then ate the skin off the rest of them. Delicious, but yikes!

- Beans and legumes
- Hemp
- Quinoa
- Yogurt
- Cheese—parmesan is one of the better choices for protein
- Nuts and seeds
- Eggs. As mentioned, I use egg whites to hit my protein goals for bodybuilding, but I highly recommend you eat that whole egg!
- Protein shakes. Use them only as a supplement. They're great for protein on the go, but if you're depending on just shakes to get your protein, you're going to run into problems. I have one right after my workout when my muscle cells are screaming for some amino acids to repair themselves, and I sometimes have one before bed. A protein shake or protein pudding can be a nice dessert.

When we think about building muscle, we often think about protein, which is absolutely correct. You do need protein to help build muscle. But just because it's necessary to build muscle does not mean it needs to be consumed in large amounts. Eat too much and you're just wasting money and possibly damaging your health. Protein, along with all healthy foods and lifestyle habits, should never be taken to extremes.

Eat the correct amount for your body, activity level, and goals, and you will get results.

★

Here's what you're "supposed" to do:
Eat 0.8 to 1 gram of protein
per pound of body weight.

★

Here's what I did:
I decided that protein must be fattening,
so I became a vegetarian for a while.
I eliminated all meat and only ate carbs because
I heard that vegetarians were always thin.

★

How that worked out for me:
I gained weight when I tried to be vegetarian.
If you do it right and get enough protein,
being vegetarian can be super healthy. I just didn't
know enough about plant-based protein sources to

do it well, so instead of becoming super healthy
I became tired and weak and gained weight.

★

What are you going to do?

The "C" Word: Carbs
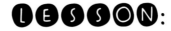**:**

Carbs aren't bad, it's the type of carbs you eat that will determine how healthy you are. Choose natural sources of carbs, not processed.

Not all carbs are bad for you, but unfortunately, there are a lot of processed carbs being disguised as healthy foods that are wreaking havoc in your body. Natural carbs are essential to good health (for more information, see the Resources section), while processed carbs assist in weight gain. Some people are unaware of the difference between healthy and unhealthy carbs.

Here's why you need carbs:

Energy. Your body's preferred source of energy is carbohydrates. Your body can switch over to fats if absolutely necessary (like when following a keto-style diet), but its preferred source is carbs. When I'm preparing for a competition and trying to put on muscle, I increase my carb intake so I have the energy to perform the exercises needed.

Good mood. Carbs promote the production of serotonin, our feel-good brain chemical.

Heart health. Including foods such as oatmeal and beans in your diet have been shown to lower LDL (our bad cholesterol). People who eat whole grains tend to have higher HDL (our good cholesterol) and lower LDL.

Brain function. Your brain will operate more optimally when you include healthy carbs in your diet.

Satisfaction. The fiber found in healthy carbohydrate foods makes you feel fuller and satiated.

So, what exactly are healthy carbs and where do you find them? And which carbs are unhealthy, and how can you avoid their tempting call?

Healthy carbs are plants, root vegetables, and whole grains that have been minimally processed. If you're not sure how to tell how processed a grain is, review the cooking times. If your oatmeal can be ready in three minutes, it's over processed. Oats should take about twenty minutes to cook. If your carbs are white and didn't come out of the ground white, they're over processed. For instance, white rice is more processed than brown rice.

Also, be sure to look at the ingredient list. There are some clever marketing techniques that make unhealthy foods sound good for you. The ingredient list should be short (about five ingredients). You should be able to recognize all the ingredients as actual food that came from the earth; plus, there should be no added sugars (any word that ends in "ose" is a sugar) or syrups, even if they are listed as "raw" or "natural." Raw and natural sugars/syrups are just sugar. (Note: If you do need a sweetener, use raw honey or pure maple syrup, but minimize your use because these are still sugars. However, they have other nutrients as well as enzymes you need in order for your body to use them as energy as opposed to storing them as fat.)

Your healthy carbs mostly live on the perimeter of the grocery store. Unhealthy carbs are the ones you find in the junk food aisle, the cereal aisle, and (for the most part) the bread aisle. If you want bread, go to the refrigerated section and look for sprouted grain bread. To avoid the tempting call of unhealthy carbs, stick to the perimeter of the grocery store.

★

Here's what you're "supposed" to do:
Eat healthy carbs in their natural form.

★

Here's what I did:
I ate healthy carbs and tried to avoid
processed carbs as much as possible.

★

How that worked out for me:
It would have worked out fine, but because
I was restricting my calorie intake so much,
I got intense cravings for processed carbs and
eventually binged on them.

★

What are you going to do?

Sugar, Sugar

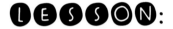

**Processed sugar will destroy your health,
as it causes physical and mental issues.
The only sugar that's suitable for consumption
on a regular basis is naturally occurring sugars
in their natural, unprocessed form.**

When I looked back at the food I ate growing up, I realized that I had sugar at every single meal. For breakfast, we normally had cereal like Rice Crispies, Corn Flakes, and Puffed Wheat. While not considered "sugary" cereals, they do have a bit of sugar in them. And because I had a sweet tooth, I added layers of white sugar to them. By the time I got to the bottom of the bowl, the leftover milk was super sweet. It still makes my mouth water to think about it. Our lunch was usually a sandwich with a processed cheese product (there's not enough actual cheese in those processed slices for it to be called "cheese"), some sort of sliced meat product, margarine, Miracle Whip (which is loaded with sugar), and sometimes sweet mustard (the sweet means it has sugar in it). We had fruit with our sandwiches, so we did eat some healthy sugar. Our snacks were typically some delicious baked goodies that my mom made (she loved to bake for us, and we loved to eat her treats!).

Our dinner consisted of meat, potatoes, and vegetables that I would drown in ketchup (there's lots of sugar in ketchup). And there was usually some sort of dessert because I had an insatiable sweet tooth.

Little did I know at the time that sugar causes so many problems (visit the Resources section for additional information). Sugar:

Can cause weight gain. You can eat a large amount of sugar without feeling full. And sometimes sugary treats actually make you crave more, resulting in consuming way too many calories that will lead to weight gain. Did you know that some obese people are actually malnourished? It's because they're eating a lot of calories from food that is lacking nutrients.

May increase your risk of heart disease. Sugar causes widespread inflammation in your body and inflammation is the root of all disease, including heart disease.

Increases your risk for type 2 diabetes. Eating sugar causes your body to release insulin and insulin is what keeps your blood sugar in check by delivering sugar to the cells that need it for energy. If you are constantly eating sugar, your body keeps releasing more and more insulin, causing your cells to become resistant to it. Thus, insulin is no longer able to do its job properly and instead of sugar being used for energy by your cells, it gets stored as fat.

Has been linked to acne. Sugar can increase androgen secretion, oil production, and inflammation, which can lead to acne.

May increase your risk of cancer. Cancer cells can only survive if they're provided with sugar. This is why a keto diet is sometimes used to help get cancer under control.

May increase your risk of depression. Sugar was probably a huge part of my struggle with depression. When I do indulge in sugar, I'm guaranteed to feel anxious and depressed the next day. Depending on the size of the indulgence, I may feel this way for two or three days. Confession: sometimes when I indulge in sugar, it is an all-out binge. I feel like I can't control myself. I'm talking putting-on-the-eatin'-pants-and-closing-the-blinds kind of bingeing. It's fun in the moment, but I always regret the sugar hangover.

May accelerate the skin-aging process. Wrinkles!

Can increase cellular aging. That means you age faster!

Drains your energy. If you are/were a sugar addict, you're probably all too familiar with the sugar high followed by the sugar low.

Can lead to fatty liver. Usually, fatty liver is associated with alcohol consumption, but sugar causes it too. There are children out there suffering from fatty liver!

As an adult, I learned more about sugar and how detrimental it was to my overall health. It causes chronic inflammation, which is known as the root of all disease. So, my first big change was cutting out sugar. It wasn't easy for me or the people around me. I had cravings, and I was cranky, but I stuck with it. One day during a spin class I realized that I had forgotten to take my Ventolin but my breathing was fine! (I used to take Ventolin before exercising so I wouldn't have an asthma attack. An easy walk could trigger my asthma, so I always had Ventolin on me.) That was a big lightbulb moment for me. Doctors used to have me on medications to try and control my asthma. They worked when I had an acute attack, but I still had asthma. The medication made it manageable but did nothing to cure it. Cutting out sugar made my asthma and other assorted allergies go away! Asthma is basically inflammation in your lungs. Sugar = inflammation! Inflammation = disease! I cut out sugar and most of my issues just disappeared.

I also noticed that my mood improved when I no longer consumed sugar. Did you know that sugar has been linked to depression? I no longer felt that heavy sense of dread that had been a normal part of my life. Life was slowly getting better for me. I saw hope, and I was ready to keep going toward it. (Note: if you are currently taking antidepressants, please consult your doctor before making any changes to your medication intake.)

Cutting out sugar literally changed my life. It was one of the best things I've ever done for myself. I need to mention here, though, that you do have to be careful when it comes to cutting something completely out of your diet. Extreme actions rarely work in the long term. As we've already seen, one extreme that became popular was to cut out all fat. Another extreme that the diet scene adopted was cutting out all sugar. And not just processed sugar, but anything with sugar, even fruit! Keto diets suddenly became so popular that there were even drinks developed that were designed to put your body into ketosis. A typical keto diet is about 5 to 10 percent net carbs (the amount of carbs minus the grams of fiber in a food), 20 to 25 percent protein, and 70 to 80 percent fat. I have nothing against keto diets. I know some people who do really well on them, and there are some pretty exciting health benefits for people with cancer and even epilepsy (see the Resources section). I do think that it is way too restrictive for the average person, however, and it can make social gatherings that are centered around food tricky. Eating should be a social activity where you share food and time with people you love. But by eating something separate from everyone else, you are isolating yourself, even though you are in a group.

So, what's a person to do about sugar? It's simple! Get your sugar from natural whole foods. But if it's a prepared food, beware. Make sure to read labels because quite often there's sugar in things you wouldn't even think it's in such as pasta sauces, salad dressings, and "healthy" cereals.

If you have the sugar monkey on your back, you need to get rid of it. And this is coming from a girl who was a straight-up sugar junkie for a huge part of her life! It's not an easy process, and the first three days are usually the worst. Do I still love/crave sugary treats? Yes! Do I indulge? I do, but I make sure not to do it very often. Persevere and get through it! I promise that it's worth it.

I challenge you to start cutting out sugar today. Promise to hang on for one full week. If that seems like too much, just promise to get through one day without processed sugar. As your mind starts to clear and you start feeling more energetic, you'll realize how much damage sugar does to your body and mind. You can totally do this!

★

Here's what you're "supposed" to do:
Limit/eliminate processed sugar. Eat natural sugars in their natural state. Steer clear of sugary, processed foods and food-like substances.

★

Here's what I did:
I ate all the sugar all the time.

★

How that worked out for me:
I was chubby, asthmatic, had bad allergies, and developed polycystic ovary syndrome. Cutting way down on sugar actually cured my asthma and allergies and has greatly improved my PCOS.

★

What are you going to do?

The Magic of Water

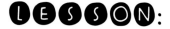:

Your body absolutely needs water to be able to function properly. Your quality of life depends on getting proper hydration.

A lot of people greatly underestimate the importance of drinking water. Most people are chronically dehydrated and don't even know it. Achy joints, fuzzy brain, inability to concentrate, inability to lose weight, adult-onset asthma, and many more issues can all be due to chronic dehydration. Who would have thought? Water is colorless and tasteless yet does so much magic in the body.

How much water should you be drinking? I tell my clients to aim for about 3 liters a day. Or you can aim to drink 1 ounce of water per pound of body weight. If you drink very little water right now, plan to ease into this increase. Start by adding one extra 8-ounce glass per day until you're comfortable with that, then continue adding slowly until you've got your hydration up to a healthy amount.

If you're looking for a way to measure whether you're drinking enough, look at the color of your urine. If it's quite dark and you haven't just taken B vitamins, you're most likely dehydrated. You want a pale yellow, like the color of straw. If your urine is clear, you're probably drinking a bit too much water.

A word of caution: there is something known as water intoxication. Basically, it's when you've drunk too much water and you've actually diluted your electrolytes to a dangerous level. People who experience it feel like they're a bit drunk, and it could lead to seizures and even death. A good rule is to not drink more than a liter per hour. (I once experienced water intoxication. Part of my prep for stage is to over hydrate for a while, so I decided to drink a whole liter of water in one sitting. I just wanted to get it down. Afterward, I felt dizzy. I got a bit panicky because I knew that I had done something wrong, so I sat still on the couch and waited for it to pass. It finally did, and I never tried guzzling a liter of water in one sitting again.)

I hope this isn't overwhelming for you. Make small changes that you're comfortable with making and don't worry about the rest until you feel ready for it. This is your journey, and the best way to be successful is to go at a pace that feels right for you. Be patient and kind to yourself, and don't forget to celebrate the victories!

★

Here's what you're "supposed" to do:
Drink about 1 ounce of water per pound
of body weight.

★

Here's what I did:
I drank at least 3 liters of water per day
(more when I'm getting ready to compete).

★

How that worked out for me:
Great! At first, I was having to run to the washroom
far too often for my liking, but my body adapted.

★

What are you going to do?

MOVING YOUR BODY!

For me, physical education class was an exercise in humiliation.

I have never been good at sports . . . like, none of them. When I was growing up, PE class always focused on some sort of sport—volleyball, field hockey, baseball, basketball, and the absolute worst one, dodgeball—and I SUCKED at all of them! And because kids are jerks, my classmates made sure I knew just how much I sucked. I wasn't chosen last for teams; I was assigned to the unlucky team that needed one more person.

The PE classes that didn't focus on sports were set up as the most terrifying playground/obstacle courses you could imagine. We had to climb ropes, balance on things that were high up, and perform other death-defying feats for the hour that was PE, a.k.a. HELL. I was chubby, asthmatic, and uncoordinated. Add these traits to my super-early metamorphosis into the first girl in her class to start developing breasts and you had what was the most traumatic school experience of my life. For me, physical activity meant changing in front of the other girls who all made fun of me for having boobies (which unfortunately stopped growing shortly after they started growing) and then either feeling humiliated by my lack of hand–eye coordination or terrified that I was going to hurt myself.

I did anything and everything to get out of physical activity. I told the teacher I forgot my gym strip, or that my asthma was bothering me, or that I had an upset stomach, and when I started my period at age eleven, I used that as an excuse. This last one was great with the male teachers—I'd just say I was having female issues and they excused me without asking any questions.

Then one day we had a guest PE teacher, the mother of one of my classmates. She was an aerobics instructor. It was my first-ever aerobics class, and I loved it! I was actually kind of good at it! We only ever had that one class with her, but it ignited a small spark in me that made me think that maybe all physical activity wasn't all that horrible.

It was years later when I went to my first aerobics class at the local recreation center. Once again it made me feel good about myself and realize that I didn't actually hate physical activity. I still remember that first class: women twenty and thirty years older than I was were dancing around like it was nothing while I was sweating and wheezing in the back row. But for once in my life no one made me feel shame about my lack of skill. Instead, these ladies encouraged me to keep coming back, so I did. Before long I was the one in the front of the class inspiring those who were struggling. Soon, physical activity became the best part of my day rather than the worst part.

Okay! We've talked about setting goals and healthy nutrition. Now, let's dive into some physical stuff! We're going to talk about finding the best fitness regime for you as well as the importance of sleeping well and practicing breathwork.

How to Start Your Fitness Journey

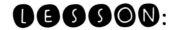:

You need to move that body!
**You need to find something that you enjoy doing
so you can happily make physical activity a
consistent and enjoyable part of your life.**

I think most of us can relate to starting and stopping something we thought we really wanted to work on. There were many times when I started a diet and fitness plan only to find myself quitting not too much later.

It's not your fault! You just need to take the right steps to ensure that you start something that will become a solid part of your life.

Here are some tips to help set you up for success:

First, attach your workout to something you already do every day. This is where you'll be taking real action, so you need to make sure it fits in your day.

Attach your workout time to something you do already. For instance, if you drop your kids off at 9 a.m. for school, make your next stop the gym. Either find a gym/studio that has a 9:30 a.m. class, hire a trainer for that time, or go to the gym on your own right after the kids start school for the day (just make sure you have a clear plan to follow so you're not just wandering around the gym wondering what to do). The key here is to fit in your workout at a time that makes sense to the rest of your day. If you are stressed about fitting in your workout, you'll end up finding an excuse not to do it.

Next, make it nonnegotiable. Make workouts a "must-do" part of your day, not a "should-do" part, or worse, a "should-try-to-fit-it-in" part of your day.

Make your workout a nonnegotiable time of your day. You wouldn't skip brushing your teeth just because you don't feel like doing it. When you make something a "must-do," you will find a way to get it done. Think about the things you do every day no matter what. A lot of those tasks are probably not very exciting or enjoyable, but you still find a way to get them done because you believe that they have to get done no matter what. Start thinking the same way about your workouts. If you're struggling, go back to the previous tip.

And finally, reward yourself. Let's face it: working out causes discomfort in the moment. In order to make something a new habit, there has to be something pleasurable about it.

Reward yourself with something! In the beginning it might need to be something exciting like a new workout outfit or new shoes. After a while, once your workouts become a habit, you can reward yourself simply by giving yourself five minutes to really focus on your gratitude for being able to use your body the way you do and feel strong and healthy. Find some sort of positive reinforcement to build momentum.

It really can be tough to talk yourself into working out. Our days are busy and working out can feel like just another chore you have to do, but maybe you can change your mindset and actually start looking forward to your workouts. Remember being a kid and getting excited about going to the playground to run around and have fun? Treat your workouts like a trip to the playground. Look at your workouts as your opportunity to have fun moving your body!

Get out there and play!

★

Here's what you're "supposed" to do:
All the steps mentioned above.

★

Here's what I did:
All the steps mentioned above.

★

How that worked out for me:
I reached my initial goal and went on
to reach more goals.

★

What are you going to do?

HIIT or Steady State—Which Is Better?

ⓛⒺⓈⓈⓄⓃ:

The best exercise is the exercise you're willing to do consistently. Consistent + persistent = success!

(Note: You must talk to your doctor before starting any exercise program! Safety first!)

The great debate! Steady state cardio or high-intensity interval training (HIIT)?

There are definitely benefits to both. I'm not going to go into the science behind the methods because it's a bit boring and both are beneficial. I will give a brief explanation of them, however, so you have an understanding of them.

Steady state cardio is the type of cardio where you engage in it for a longer period of time. When doing steady state, you work at an intensity that you can maintain for the full cardio session. Steady state is great for improving endurance because to improve at something you need to practice exactly what you're trying to improve. Steady state is also great for when you just want to tune out and enjoy some time to yourself. It can be especially magical when you do it outdoors in nature. I used to really love going for a long run even though I am truly not a runner.

HIIT is when you incorporate high-intensity intervals into your workout. These intervals are meant to be so hard that you can barely maintain the effort for thirty seconds. One of the great benefits of HIIT training is it can be done in a very short amount of time if you're pushing the intervals hard enough. For instance, instead of running at a steady state for an hour, you can do intervals where you push as hard as you can and then recover while burning about the same number of calories in about half the time. Ideally, you want to feel like you can't quite hold the intensity for thirty seconds because it's so hard. Please note that HIIT may not be a safe option for anyone new to exercise or with certain health issues that could be aggravated by pushing your body that hard.

In order to do HIIT, you need to know your body well and know when the discomfort from the exercise is good discomfort or bad discomfort. This is not to say that beginners cannot do HIIT, they just need to experiment a bit to see how hard they can push themselves safely. I've taught a few spin classes where someone new tried a class, went too hard too fast, and ended up throwing up as a result. If you've been training for a while and you know you can safely push yourself to that high discomfort level, you may be wondering how to know if you've pushed hard enough. I tell my clients to use their rate of recovery to make that determination. It should take you twice as long as the interval to recover. So, if you do a thirty-second high-intensity interval, it should take you at least a minute before you feel ready to push yourself again. If you do a thirty-second high-intensity effort and then after thirty seconds of rest you feel ready to hit it hard again, you probably didn't push your interval enough. This balance takes a bit of experimenting, though. Even fit people can push themselves to the point of throwing up if they go too hard.

If you're asking yourself whether you should do HIIT or steady state, the real question you should be asking is which one are you willing to do consistently? If I told someone that HIIT was the answer and they hated interval training, they would probably jump all in for about a week, maybe two. After that they'd be dreading their workouts and hating me, and their fitness journey could very well come to an end. And who among us hasn't gone all in with something that was pure torture on the off chance that it was the answer to our fitness dreams? How did that end? Not well probably.

Ideally, you'll have a mix of both types of exercise. I advise steady state on most days, with one or two days of HIIT thrown in. This schedule provides more variety, and more variety is what usually keeps people interested.

When I started going to the gym, I went purely to lose weight. I wanted the fat gone! I thought the only way to do that was to do endless cardio. I'd get on that damn Stairmaster and go for as long as possible, then move onto the next cardio machine. I hated my workouts! I dreaded my workouts! The only thing that kept me going was the hope that I would finally lose the weight! Then one day I asked myself what the point of it was. What should have been a fun part of my day turned into something I just didn't want to do.

When I realized that I hated cardio machines with a blind passion, I started looking at other options for working out. There was a boxing class that I always wanted to try, so I did. I was really nervous and felt super intimidated, but it seemed better to me than facing the cardio machines. After my first class, I was hooked! The same thing happened with spin. When I took my first spin class, I got nauseated and hyperventilated. I don't know what it was about that experience, but for some reason it left me wanting more!

In the end, I did boxing, aerobics, spin, and boot-camp-style classes, and I got excited about my workouts again. I also added weight training. I looked forward to my workouts, and my body composition changed. I soon became a spin instructor, and it's my absolute favorite class to teach. When people tell me that they don't like spin, I always think to myself, *But you haven't tried my spin class.* I'm not bragging, but the passion I have for teaching spin makes my classes something else! I'm getting excited just writing about it!

So, what's the point of all this? The best exercise is the exercise you know you'll do consistently because you enjoy it. Your workouts don't even need to be conventional. Maybe you have a job where you're on your feet all day, lifting boxes and doing all sorts of active tasks. Guess what? That's your workout! Maybe you love golf or some other sport. How about chasing after your kids? Don't get caught up in what you think working out "should" be. Find the activities that bring you joy. Being consistent and persistent is the key to any exercise program, so you need to know what that is for you.

What activities do you love? Maybe you don't have an answer right now. If you had asked me that question when I was a kid, I would have said there was nothing active that I liked to do. If that's you, let me ask you this: What activity have you always wanted to try?

Make a list and start doing them!

★

Here's what you're "supposed" to do:
Find physical activity that you enjoy and
look forward to so you stay consistent
and find joy in moving your body.

★

Here's what I did:
When I first started working out, I did workouts
that I didn't enjoy in the hopes that I would
lose weight and finally be happy.

★

How that worked out for me:
Not good. My workouts became something
I dreaded, and it just got harder and harder to talk
myself into doing them. Once I found activities
I enjoyed, I found myself actually getting excited
about my workout time. Some days my
workout was the best part of my day!

★

What are you going to do?

Get Your Rest to Be Your Best!

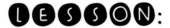 LESSON:

Sleep is imperative for a healthy mind and body. Working more and sleeping less is not a badge of honor.

Getting proper sleep allows you to function at your best. Proper sleep is really the cornerstone of our health. It has to be quality sleep, though. You could be in bed for eight hours and still wake up feeling off if those hours were not quality sleep hours.

Here are some facts about sleep that you may not be aware of:

Sleep is good for your heart and blood-vessel health. When you sleep, certain hormones are released that help with the proper function of your heart and blood vessels. If you don't get enough sleep, these hormones are not released.

Lack of sleep can affect your blood sugar levels, leaving you at higher risk for developing type 2 diabetes.

Lack of sleep will cause your body to release stress hormones, making you feel anxious and unable to make well-thought-out decisions.

When you don't get enough sleep, your immune system takes a hit. This can cause inflammation, and chronic inflammation can lead to ulcers, dementia, and even heart disease.

Lack of sleep can make you feel hungrier. Quite often when people are sleep deprived, they reach for unhealthy, sugar-filled foods in hopes of getting a bit of energy. This can easily lead to unwanted weight gain.

Lack of sleep can result in balance issues, leaving you at higher risk of falls and injuries.

Memory can be affected if you're not getting enough sleep. Deep sleep is important for memory.

Sleep is when your body repairs itself. If you find that you don't feel like you're recovering well from your workouts, it could be from lack of sleep (visit the Resources section for more information).

It took me a long time to realize the importance of sleep and make it a priority. I used to teach 6 a.m. classes, so I was always up early. I wasn't disciplined enough to get to bed early, however, and I drank wine every night. Alcohol, even just a drink or two, absolutely decreases the quality of your sleep. It might help you fall asleep, or pass out, but the quality of sleep is poor. I really noticed this when I started competing in bodybuilding and had to cut my drinking from every night to just one night a week. That first morning I woke up after not drinking the night before was amazing! It was enough to convince me that I really didn't need my nightly wine.

Here are some things I now do to get a quality night's sleep:

I put on blue-light–canceling glasses about thirty minutes to an hour before I plan on going to bed (see the Resources section for more information). Blue light is emitted from devices such as smartphones, computers, and televisions. Blue light has the same light spectrum as daylight, so if you're looking at your device after it's gotten dark, your brain thinks it's still daylight and doesn't produce the sleep hormones that normally get produced as a reaction to nighttime. I got my glasses from Amazon. Make sure you get ones that actually work. Be ready to spend more than $20.

I take magnesium as part of my bedtime routine. Magnesium helps you relax. From what I've learned, magnesium glycinate is a very absorbable form of magnesium. Just a note here: just because some is good does not mean that more is better. If you overdo magnesium, it can cause diarrhea.

I put in earplugs. I'm sensitive to noise.

I keep the bedroom dark and cool.

I sleep with a sleep mask to block out any light that might be in my room.

I practice the same sleep routine every night and have no problem falling asleep or staying asleep, and I naturally wake up about seven to eight hours after going to bed. Keeping your bedtime routine consistent is really the trick for quality sleep. As soon as I begin the first part of my routine, I can feel my body and mind relaxing because I've trained my brain to recognize it as shutting down for the night. I feel amazing!

Getting enough sleep is paramount to good health. If you're trying to increase your sleep, try going to bed just fifteen minutes earlier than usual. Once you get comfortable with going to bed fifteen minutes earlier, try thirty minutes earlier. Keep taking small steps until you're getting the amount of sleep you need.

★

Here's what you're "supposed" to do:
Get between seven and nine hours of
quality sleep every night.

★

Here's what I did:
Stayed up late, drank, and then slept for a
few hours before I got up to teach the first
of up to four spin classes a day.

★

How that worked out for me:
I was exhausted and usually grouchy.
I definitely was not able to give 100 percent of
myself to my class participants and clients. Looking
back, I realize that I was being very selfish.

★

What are you going to do?

Just Breathe

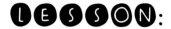:

Breathwork works!

Do you ever pay attention to your breathing? Luckily for us, breathing is an automatic function so we don't actually have to think about it to make it happen, but great things can occur when we do take time each day to focus on breathing.

Most people breathe quite shallowly throughout their day. Shallow and quick breathing, especially through your mouth, activates the sympathetic nervous system, which is your fight-or-flight system. Thus, most people are spending their time in what feels like crisis mode for their body. This causes a cascade of hormonal reactions that can leave you in chronic stress, which will slowly break you down.

I remember when I was a teenager and my mom had me see a psychologist to help me deal with my stress. The psychologist suggested practicing breathwork. I didn't take it seriously at the time, so I didn't do it. How could simple breathing possibly help me? I really wish that I had been more open and tried it out then. I probably would have saved myself a lot of discomfort and anxiety. It wasn't until I first tried yoga that I finally felt what it was like to control my own stress by simply breathing.

Try taking a few deep breaths right now. Inhale through your nose until you feel your chest and belly expand, then slowly let that breath out through your mouth. Go ahead, do it.

How do you feel?

Inhaling deeply and slowly and then exhaling slowly activates the parasympathetic nervous system (also known as your rest and digest system). By breathing deeply, you're telling your brain and body that everything is okay and there is no need to fight or flee.

Deep breathing has an instantly calming effect. Here is my favorite breath practice:

Inhale through your nose for a count of four. Hold that breath for a count of seven, then exhale through your mouth for a count of eight. Repeat four times.

I do this exercise at night when I go to bed. I also try to remember to do it before I eat so my body is ready to digest in a relaxed state. If I'm feeling overly stressed for any reason, I do it then too. The great thing about it is that you can do it anywhere. Stuck in traffic and feeling like you're about to explode? Try the breathwork I just explained (see the Resources section for more information). No one can tell that you're doing it, and it puts you in a calm state of mind so you can deal with the stress you're feeling. I know it might sound too simple to be true, but I want you to give it a try. Try doing the breathing exercise at least once a day to start.

★

Here's what you're "supposed" to do:
Use breathwork to help control your stress.

★

Here's what I did:
When I finally opened myself up to the possibility of it working, I started practicing it on a regular basis.

★

How that worked out for me:
Great! Things that used to be really stressful didn't seem as colossal anymore. When I was having problems falling asleep, doing my breathwork helped me. I felt so powerful because I finally realized that I really do have the power to control how I view and react to the world.

★

What are you going to do?

CONCLUSION
❤

♡

FROM HOT MESS TO HAPPINESS

This book tells the story of how I went from a hot mess to happiness.

Happiness isn't limited to everyone else. It isn't limited to all those people who seem to have their life together. But I used to think that it was. I used to think that being happy was slated into some sort of exclusive club that I didn't have access to.

I still remember how I felt at my breaking point, my rock bottom. I had the day off, so I slept late. When I woke up, I had the same anxious feeling I experienced whenever I had a day that didn't include a specific schedule to follow. I was depressed and anxious and felt lost, so I soothed myself with leftover Chinese food. Once I was done eating, however, the feeling of comfort turned into self-loathing. I went back to bed and tried to sleep for as long as possible so I didn't have to deal with the feelings.

When I woke up, I felt even worse. I felt weak for giving in to my craving, and I was bloated, depressed, and anxious. This was not a new experience for me, though. It was a habit that had become a part of my life. I don't know why, but on that particular day I just decided that I'd had enough of starving myself and then bingeing and hating myself on a level that I can't even explain fully with words. I felt pain to a degree that I hadn't acknowledged before.

On that fateful morning I thought to myself, *Screw it! I'm going to try taking care of myself by eating properly!* I decided that if it resulted in weight gain, I could always go back to my previous lifestyle. It was a bargain I had with myself.

My life changed that day, but not right away. It took a lot of effort and massive action, but I had gotten to that pain point that I could no longer tolerate. I felt like I would rather be dead than keep living the way I had been. It may sound a tad dramatic, but that's how I felt.

You can feel like you're a complete hot mess and still be able to come out on top. Just because you're a hot mess right now doesn't mean you are doomed to be unhappy. You too can change for the better and live the life you want, and you don't have to be a superhero to do it. Simplicity is key. You need to stop overthinking, stop trying to figure out how you don't measure up, and stop trying to figure out what everyone wants from you. You need to just live your life in a way that feels authentic. Stop trying to figure out how to make everyone around you happy. You can't please everyone all the time.

You have complete control over your life, how you live it, and how you feel about yourself. You can change everything, and the good news is, it's quite achievable. A few shifts in thinking and a few realistic lifestyle changes are all you need to completely flip your life and find the joy in being you.

Be Open to the Lessons

Everyone has the ability to live a self-empowered life. You can change your mindset and take life as it comes, then take note of the lessons that come along with it.

You need to accept the changes and setbacks that happen, though. If you fight the lessons, you get stuck in feeling sorry for yourself and won't leave any room for happiness, growth, and self-acceptance. Remember that the experiences you have, good and bad, are what shape and strengthen you. Rather than being bitter about the bad and complaining about them, you have to find the lesson so you can move forward.

Here are some of the most important lessons I've outlined in this book:

Make friends with yourself. Before you can really love and enjoy life, you need to make peace with yourself and become your own best friend.

Keep a positive mindset. This one's not always easy but if you really search, then you can find something positive in almost any situation. Once you learn to live in a positive mindset, life becomes much more enjoyable.

Find your passion. We all have something that we absolutely love to do. It would be a shame to waste the opportunity to live in your happy place. Not only do you miss out, but others may be missing out on a beautiful gift that only you can deliver.

Set goals for yourself. If you don't have goals you may become stagnant, then life becomes nothing but a never-ending chore.

Nourish your body. The only way to have a healthy mind is to nourish your body.

Find a physical activity that you love. Never in a million years did I think I'd ever like physical activity, but once I found something that I enjoyed doing, I couldn't believe I was ever able to live happily without it.

Get enough sleep. Do not underestimate the power of proper sleep. Sleep is when your body and mind repair and rebuild. Without proper sleep everything starts to fall apart. If you want to function at a high level and keep yourself healthy, you have to get proper sleep.

These lessons are simple, but just because something is simple does not mean it's easy. Allow yourself to surrender to the simplicity and, even when it's hard, do it knowing that the payoff is going to be 100 percent worth the effort.

Happiness Ahead!

As a teenager I loved looking at fitness magazines. I'd see pictures of the women competing on stage and think about how beautiful they were. I had gotten into weight training and learned that I put on muscle quite easily, so there was a tiny part of me that thought maybe I'd be able to compete one day.

I've always been a strong girl, so I really enjoyed challenging myself with weights. My body started to change, and I began receiving compliments on my physique! People often told me that they wished they had legs like mine! But quite often it was men who told me this, so of course I took that to mean that I looked masculine. (I was always so quick to jump to the negative when it came to my body.) I kept weight training, though, because I loved it, but I battled the idea that I was too big and masculine looking. It wasn't until I entered my forties that I really and truly embraced my muscular legs and felt at peace with the fact that I'm a muscular girl. I wish that I had embraced my muscular body sooner.

Bodybuilding sounds like the last thing that a person with a history of self-hate and eating disorders should do. If I knew someone who struggled with an eating disorder and they said they were thinking about trying it, I'd advise them not to. When it comes to myself, however, I tend to want to do things people tell me I shouldn't. Before I started bodybuilding and competing, I was curious about whether I could do it. I knew my head was in the right place because I was motivated to put myself out there in total discomfort. I didn't get into it because I felt like I had to win, and I knew that if I didn't win it wasn't because I wasn't good enough. I honestly just wanted a challenge. I had the raw material—muscle and determination—and the thought of doing something that scared me was exhilarating. I felt like I had a new purpose.

Fast-forward to forty-three, and I finally got on stage. That's right, forty-three! I truly believe that if I had tried it in my twenties or thirties, it would have really messed me up. But when I reached forty, I started feeling more comfortable with myself. Now, I've placed within the top four in all my competitions. In my fourth competition I placed second in Grandmasters (forty-five and older) and Masters (thirty-five and older—I was forty-six!). In my fifth competition I finally earned first place in Masters. In my sixth, I placed first in Open (all ages) and second in Masters and Grandmasters. I plan to keep competing because I love it and I now feel comfortable enough in my body. Competing makes me feel powerful and proud.

For much of my life I was laser-focused on one goal: I wanted nothing more than to look and act how I thought society wanted me to look and act so I would be accepted and loved. I had let my interpretation of the messages I received rule my life and trap me in a tiny and stifling box. When I hit my rock bottom, I was desperate to be happy and realized that what I was doing wasn't working no matter how many times I tried doing it. Insanity truly is doing the same thing over and over and expecting different results.

So, what are you doing now? Have you fallen into the trap of doing the same things and expecting the results you so desperately want only to fall short? Are you living a life that is frustrating and maybe even self-destructive? Are you ready for a change for the better?

My journey to being happy and fulfilled started with one small, simple change. It was not at all easy for me, but it was simple enough to make it doable. Once I made that small change, the momentum started! Once I felt comfortable with that small, simple change, I added another doable action. I kept adding small, simple changes until it became comfortable, and the result was happiness. I had called an end to my internal war and became focused on making life better for myself. The key for me was to be consistent in my effort, and to be consistent meant keeping things small and simple instead of always going to extremes. It meant patience and kindness. It meant becoming friends with myself and treating myself with the love and respect I needed and deserved.

Growing up, I was a hot mess. In early adulthood, I was a hot mess. I still have my moments, but for the most part, I am truly happy. I slowly learned who I was and what I wanted for my life. I slowly learned to accept and actually be comfortable with myself instead of looking at and listening to everyone else. Life has lessons, and if you let them, those lessons will lead you from being a hot mess to finding true happiness.

RESOURCES

Taking Steps to Clean Up the Hot Mess

For information and support regarding eating disorders, see the website for ANAD (the National Association of Anorexia Nervosa and Associated Disorders). Did you know that eating disorders affect at least 9 percent of the population worldwide, and that less than 6 percent of people with eating disorders are medically diagnosed as "underweight"? (https://anad.org/eating-disorders-statistics)

Making Friends with Yourself

For more on the genetic component of depression (and for more on depression generally), visit this link at MedicinePlus: https://medlineplus.gov/genetics/condition/depression/#inheritance.

Learn to Be Present

For more on Eckhart Tolle and his writing, visit his website: https://eckharttolle.com/.

Find the Lesson in the Struggle

For more "Success Secrets" from Wayne Dyer, visit https://www.drwaynedyer.com/blog/success-secrets/.

It All Starts with Food

Visit Cory Holly's website here: http://www.coryholly.com/.

Visit Shawn Stevenson's *The Model Health Show* here: https:// themodelhealthshow.com/.

Foods That Talk

What's a calorie? "The calorie was originally defined as the amount of heat required at a pressure of 1 standard atmosphere to raise the temperature of 1 gram of water 1° Celsius" (https:// www.britannica.com/science/calorie).

My (Partial) Breakup with Alcohol

For more on the effects of alcohol on muscle growth, visit https://blog.nasm.org/does-alcohol-affect-muscle-growth.

The "F" Word: Fat Is Not the Enemy

For more on the obesity pandemic, visit https://www.ncbi.nlm. nih.gov/books/NBK44656/.

For more about healthy fats, visit https://www.healthline.com/ health/food-nutrition/healthy-fats-guidelines.

For more on the link between triglycerides and Alzheimer's disease, visit https://www.ncbi.nlm.nih.gov/pmc/articles/ PMC4712972/; for more on the link between triglycerides and belly fat, see https://pubmed.ncbi.nlm.nih.gov/25636220/.

Where's the Beef? Facts about Protein

For more on the link between protein and bone health, visit the following 2017 study: "Dietary protein and bone health: a systematic review and meta-analysis from the National Osteoporosis Foundation" (https://pubmed.ncbi.nlm.nih.gov/28404575/).

For more on the link between protein and blood pressure, visit the following 2003 study: "The effects of protein intake on blood pressure and cardiovascular disease" (https://pubmed.ncbi.nlm.nih.gov/12544662/).

For more on the link between protein and your kidneys, visit https://www.healthline.com/nutrition/10-reasons-to-eat-more-protein#TOC_TITLE_HDR_9.

The "C" Word: Carbs

For more on the benefits of carbohydrates, visit https://www.inlifehealthcare.com/benefits-of-eating-carbohydrates/.

Sugar, Sugar

For more on the link between keto diets and cancer, visit https://pubmed.ncbi.nlm.nih.gov/31399389/. For information on the link between keto diets and epilepsy, see https://www.ncbi.nlm.nih.gov/pmc/articles/PMC6836058/.

For more on the link between sugar and depression, visit this 2019 study: "The depressogenic potential of added dietary sugars" (https://pubmed.ncbi.nlm.nih.gov/31634771/).

For more on this and many other reasons why sugar is bad for you, visit https://www.amerimedcpr.com/11-reasons-why-too-much-sugar-is-bad-for-you/.

Get Your Rest to Be Your Best!

For more facts on sleep, visit https://www.verywellhealth.com/top-health-benefits-of-a-good-nights-sleep-2223766.

For more on blue-light glasses, visit https://thlsleep.com/blogs/sleep/test-blue-light-glasses.

Just Breathe

I learned this technique from Dr. Andrew Weil. You can learn more about it here: https://www.drweil.com/health-wellness/body-mind-spirit/stress-anxiety/breathing-three-exercises/

Manufactured by Amazon.ca
Acheson, AB

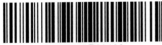